I0091122

BEFORE WE BEGIN...

I am not a medical professional, nor in any way a mental health expert. I am simply an imperfect everyday woman telling my story in the hope that it shines further light on a topic that is forever close to my heart. It is with deep sincerity and respect that I acknowledge the pain of the human psyche as downright debilitating, at times leaving us feeling isolated and helpless. If you or someone you know is struggling, **please reach out for help.** In the back of this book is a comprehensive list of professional mental health services providing immediate assistance. And beyond anything else, I want you to know that no matter how it may feel, you *can* transcend the isolation, the one and only commitment you need to make is to never *ever* give up! Em xox

Copyright © 2018 by Emma Thomson

All rights reserved. No part of this book may be
reproduced in any form or by any means, electronic or
mechanical, including photocopying, recording or by
any information or retrieval, without prior permission
in writing from the publisher. Any views and opinions
expressed herein are strictly the author's own. Thank
you for your support of the author's rights.

Originally published in 2018 by EM Corporate Group.
www.emisforyou.com.au

Grateful acknowledgment is made to Headjam Creative
Agency for the book cover & format design.
www.headjam.com.au

The publisher is not responsible for websites (or their
content) outlined within this book that are not owned
by the publisher.

ISBN 978-0-6484525-2-2

ONCE UPON INSANITY

A crazy journey of
self acceptance

by Emma Thomson

with contributions by Amy Lovat

CONTENTS

"People who wade into discomfort and vulnerability and tell the truth about their stories are the real badasses."

— BRENÉ BROWN
'RISING STRONG'

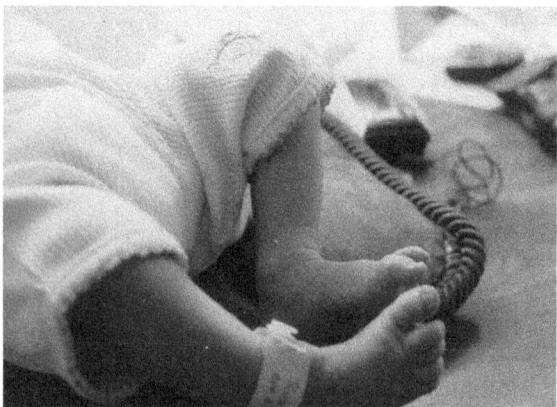

DEDICATION

To my dearest Gabriel, this book is for you.

It is a story of hope. It is what you taught me.

May the pages ahead encourage you to keep investing in the qualities of your heart, for therein lies the key beyond suffering.

Never stop sharing those gorgeous little pieces with the world.

You've got this my babe.

And to put it frankly, *thank you* just doesn't cut it.

PROLOGUE

"Welcome to hell. Read this."

She threw a book at my head and I ducked
before it smacked me in the face.
The paperback fell to the floor and I was
terrified. It didn't matter, though, because
I believed with every fibre of my being that
my mother was coming to pick me up when
she finished work at 3 o'clock. It didn't matter
that there was some strung out wiry woman
throwing shit at me in a place where I could hear
ear-splitting screaming inside my mind. Mum was
coming to rescue me. She would be here soon.

I sat cross-legged on a single bed, the first in a
row of four, all covered in sterile white sheets.
The book-throwing woman entered the room
and sat on the bed furthest from the door,
rocking back and forth like insane people do
in the movies. I looked at the clock: 11:00am.
I silently counted, only four more hours.

Here's what I didn't know at the time:

I was in a hospital for the clinically insane.

An ugly expanse of brick and concrete, otherwise known as the world's most depressing building, where the walls stained a darker brownish-grey when it rained. On the other side of the street was the scenic coastal headlands. To the left, you could see as far as the lighthouse on the peninsula, and to the right, jagged rocky cliff faces reached vertically upward from the waves crashing below. Somewhere in the middle, cafes and shops lined the esplanade, surfers practiced their ocean religion, and young lovers stole kisses beneath beach umbrellas. Polar opposite lives, divided by two lanes of traffic and a white picket fence.

I had been brought here by my father, a few hours after he began his first shift taking care of me. I required 24-hour-a-day supervision, round the clock care that by this point was definitely taking its toll on everyone. I had been diagnosed with a psychotic illness, and I was crippled with traumatic hallucinations day and night.

My brain was shattered, it was as if an atomic bomb had exploded inside my head. I was suicidal. Completely insane. And my mother was definitely not coming to pick me up at 3:00pm.

I was also not aware that I would spend the next six weeks surrounded by crazy people in a mental ward where patients and carers were almost indistinguishable from each other. I certainly didn't know that the next year of my life would see me fighting one hell of an uphill battle against the pressure to accept myself as just another mental health statistic. And I had absolutely no idea that, 20 months and 16 days from becoming a Ward of the State, I would give birth to a healthy baby boy.

TIGERS & STRIPES

CHAPTER ONE

I was never destined to be a young mum. Schizophrenics don't make the best parents. The prognosis was dyer, my life was in tatters. And yet, he arrived. A healthy baby boy with the biggest brown eyes I had ever looked into. Relaxed and content, the world at his feet. I will never forget the sense of calm that washed over me as soon as he took his first breath. How I had actually managed to bring a peaceful child into this world was beyond me. Baffling and intriguing at the same time because 'peaceful' would never *ever* have been how I would've described myself.

I always felt different. I always felt like I didn't fit in. As a child, I had a strong sense that nothing made sense, and it frightened me a lot. I attached myself to my mother from a young age, I mean physically gripped onto her, I felt that if I were to ever let go, I would literally float away. She was my safety. I was incredibly sensitive. Forever the observant one, I learned a great deal through watching others and I knew a lot, but I would only ever share what I knew in front of those whom I greatly trusted.

As a baby, it took me a long time to walk. Not because I couldn't, but because I wanted to make sure I could do it perfectly before I tried. From right back at the beginning I was frightened to fall over.

Perfectionism was my crux from the get go.

I was a deeply loving and compassionate little girl, but without a shadow of a doubt the amount of pressure I placed upon myself to be perfect had a huge bearing on my brain chemistry. My earliest of memories are littered with fear of never being good enough, and that way of thinking most certainly took its toll on those little neurons and synapses buzzing away inside my skull. One long daily battle after another of people pleasing and needing to prove myself. Exhausting. Intoxicating. And isolating. Yet something that took me years to realise that I share with many others. I've never been a lone ranger in the struggle with perfectionism. It is a battle that so many of us endure every goddamn minute of our waking lives.

I had a fairly privileged childhood. If there's such a thing as normal then I guess mine was, to a point. It was 1984 when I burst into the world three weeks early, during a fast and uncomplicated delivery. A welcome relief from the trauma my mother had suffered during my older sister's birth a few years earlier. My parents, sister and I lived on an island until I was four. It really was one of those once-in-a-lifetime opportunities; a young family living life fairly different to the norm, nestled amongst the spectacular waterway known as the Hawkesbury River. We were totally surrounded by water, and living there, it felt as if we were on holidays all of the time. I don't recall a lot from this time as I was so young, but I know my mother was close to me at all times.

From the river we moved to the mountains and the landscape was completely different — but I don't just mean the scenery. My little sister was born, my mother went back to work, and I became physically ill with anxiety when it was time for me to start school. I couldn't stand to be away from mum, she was more than my comfort zone. She was familiar and therefore safe. I felt much more secure at home. The unknown was my enemy, and school was the unknown.

In the classroom, I was as quiet as a mouse, but I didn't miss a beat. My teachers were fascinated by my ability to say nothing but understand everything. I eventually learned to love that little Catholic school. It became familiar and I began to feel safe and settled. My confidence grew enormously and I felt happy and relaxed. Then out of nowhere, with little prior warning, my parents decided to move us to a new school. Although I know it was a decision they really struggled with, I mean this kind of a call is never *easy* to make, I felt totally uprooted and confused.

We moved to the public school next door, just over the fence from that little Catholic school, and it was here where my sisters and I became known as the principal's daughters.

This move was tough. The self-confidence I had just began to grasp instantly evaporated. I wasn't good at sharing my feelings, so instead I buried them. I longed to feel safe, but I had no idea how to navigate through this vast sea of emotions. I hated that I took everything so seriously, why couldn't I just adapt? It was only across the fence for goodness sakes! No big deal at all, right? But no. It was a big deal to me. The feeling of being insecure was creeping up again. My mind was constantly buzzing and I recall often feeling dizzy. I quickly retreated and thought it best to build a wall around my little heart. If it was safety that I was seeking then feelings were definitely a no-go zone. I couldn't make sense of them and that to me was a failure. I became incredibly hard on myself. I was ten years old, tiny in stature, yet

fiercely defensive well beyond my years.
And no doubt difficult to parent.

I became a real challenge for my mother. Much more challenging than my sisters were for her. I often felt misunderstood, yet desperate to be heard at the same time. There was an intensity about me, and I seemed to not be able to help it. This full-on intensity, and my feelings of not belonging anywhere, I couldn't separate.

They went together like a tiger and stripes.

It was true I was a deeply sensitive child, and I couldn't quite put my finger on why. I remember always wishing that I wasn't like it because things didn't slide off me like they did off others, like the whole water off a duck's back thing. Instead the feelings clung to my skin, seeping under slowly and collecting in this great chasm inside.

I must admit how greatly fortunate I am to not have stories of childhood abuse and neglect that may serve to explain how I eventually became so ill. And even though no-one could pin point it at the time, there was a *reason* why I eventually lost my mind.

It was during my third-grade year that the bullying started. My older sister was bullied as well. She was in year 6 at the time and she ended up moving to an interstate boarding school to escape. I remember feeling so in awe of her for being brave enough to make that decision. I wanted to be more like her but I just couldn't fathom the idea of living away from home. I felt sick at the thought. My mother remained to be my security blanket, so instead I chose to ride out the torment.

I can't begin to describe the level of misery. Being such a small school there really was no place to hide. I felt powerless, alone and filled with self-loathing. One day I would arrive at school and the other girls would be friendly, and would present as if everything were ok. I would begin to relax a little, finally I felt as if I had been given a chance to really fit in. I'd breathe again, even start looking forward to school the next day then...BAM! The rug would be pulled out from under me and the games would begin once more. I was victimised. Totally locked out, confused and alone.

There was no doubt about it, the cracks were starting to appear. The bullying was excruciating, but nothing like the physical waves of anxiety that soon took hold.

I internalised it all, full blown anxiety which meant gut-turning nausea, a racing heart, nightmares, appetite loss, inability to concentrate, shallow breathing and nervousness that was off the charts. Something was definitely wrong, and riddled with shame, I remained silent, never discussing it at home.

It took me five long years to find the courage to stand up for myself. I'll never forget the day the torment at school stopped. I can picture the scene in my mind like it was yesterday. I only realize now in writing this, how profound a moment in my life it honestly was. I stood at the top of the stairs outside my grade 7 classroom and I confronted the girls who'd caused me endless school yard grief on and off over the years. I made it perfectly clear that I wouldn't be bullied into leaving the school, I was not going anywhere. Like it or lump it, either way, I would not be a victim anymore.

It felt like I had finally exhaled, like I was finally able to take one slow, long breath out. And then begin again. I wiped the slate clean and we all became good friends after that day. Just like the flick of a switch, we were cool. And thankfully it remained that way.

I learned very early in life that the capacity to forgive is always a strength, never a weakness.

I was now fourteen, and things were just starting to look a little brighter, when my parents decided to move towns. My father embarked on a significant career change which saw us relocate to a larger town. I was a small fish thrown into a deep sea at my new, *huge* high school — the total number of students in my year group matched the total number of students in the entirety of my previous school. It was quite the hurdle at first, the usual panic set in and I was incredibly nervous and afraid. But do you know what? After a matter of weeks, I absolutely loved it. There was something about the anonymity that I thrived on. It didn't matter that I still felt like a bit of a weirdo, that something about life on earth remained to be slightly off-putting. I found my people. Not the ultra-popular group, or the full-on emo group, or the total nerd group, but somewhere in the middle.

It was the kind of safety that I always craved. I started some great friendships, I began to learn a lot about myself, and then...

We moved again. Dad took a promotion and we moved quickly to the city by the sea. I was once again thrust into a world that I despised, awkward, deeply sensitive and this time feeling emotionally out of control. I was enrolled at a small private school and on the morning of the first day at my new school, I threw one of the most massive tantrums of my life. I made myself sick, I mean physically vomit. I was hanging onto the banister of the staircase refusing to let go. Mum was pulling at my convulsing body, attempting to pry my fingers from the timber, begging me to calm down. I was beyond anxious. Talk about dramatic behaviour I know, but the fear was crippling and I simply couldn't cope. I didn't want to go through the whole process again. To belong, to feel like I fit somewhere was all that I longed for. What if nobody liked me? The fear literally became intoxicating.

It took me a while to find my footing at this small and strongly religious school. To be honest, the strict religious rules just simply didn't fly with me. With a curious nature and an analytical brain, religion really didn't make a lot of sense. I questioned everything and I pushed the boundaries. Funny that, I still do today. At age sixteen, one thing that I can recall at school really getting to me, was the limits placed on sex education. The reason being of course that sex outside of marriage was an absolute sin according to certain belief systems. Abstinence was apparently all the sex education teenagers needed in the year 2000.

"I don't understand... I thought Jesus was friends with prostitutes?" I piped up from the back row of the classroom one day. And was promptly sent out of class.

Come to think of it, I spent a lot of time out of class actually, both physically and mentally. I was fairly outspoken, quite the frustrated teenager, and never really happy. I naturally gravitated toward rebellion and I had developed quite the bad girl streak. And at times I was angry. About what? I don't even know. But I can recall some days where it was like there was this huge fire burning inside. Of course it was housed behind the careless and cool adolescent façade I'd fashioned for myself.

For the first time, it wasn't just about my school environment, I felt like I didn't fit into my home environment either. I wanted my parent's attention. I wanted to talk about some real shit for once. The topics of relationships, hormones, drugs, alcohol, study pressure, the birds and the bees, these were all off limits. We didn't ever talk about the real shit. Our after-school activities of dance and music and maths tutoring were far more important to discuss, along with what we were having for dinner and what needed to be *done* trumped conversation surrounding feelings every day of the week. It was busy. Busy was the most important. Busy meant winning at life. But busy very soon became isolating.

Peta was away at boarding school, Han was just a kid, and there I was feeling like an alien.

My parents often seemed preoccupied, but they did their best to keep the family 'together' in the only way they knew how.

Mum *did* motherhood, but I think within herself she never felt like she was built to be a mother. It was like she had a list of checkboxes to tick off, and she was forever consumed in her own thoughts because of the continuous array of work she had on her plate. It was during my teenage years that she became even more distant, she seemed to have much more on her mind. I noticed the distance physically as well, a far cry from the days of the tiny toddler who consistently slept in her bed and was always in her arms. Mum was never big on physical affection but by now we barely even hugged each other. We had very little conversation besides the usual day to day chat, and we *never* talked about our feelings. I remember linking the idea of talking about your feelings to being that of useless conversation. Not productive at all. Lazy talk. And on the note of laziness, in our house, a sick day was actually a "stop being fat and lazy" day. There was endless busy-ness and always something to get done. No time for feelings, no space for peace. In looking back, I realise how stressful life had become, as if there was a constant buzzing electrical current surrounding our family home. It was hectic, yet oh so normal.

I threw a lot of tantrums when I was young. Looking back now I think it was due to the level of trauma I experienced in the school yard. I would lose it whenever I felt judged or misunderstood. I wasn't good with feelings because as I've made clear by now, we were very much a thought-based family. My parents were and remain to be incredibly smart people — both brilliantly capable and intelligent. The problem? Their entire self-worth was wrapped up in their ability to perform, to execute, to succeed and to do do do. Both of them were definitely workaholics. And I inherited their work ethic, plus the attached subconscious low self-worth that went with it.

When it came to problems, in our house it was always about finding solutions. "Don't let it get to you," they'd say, knives and forks paused over the Friday evening meal we shared that had become a bit of a tradition.

"Other people's opinion of you is none of your business," said my father. As if that kind of resilience nod was going to aid my pain.
I mean sure, it most certainly makes a lot more sense now. But back then, it was bullshit. And frustrating. I was the ultimate people pleaser. I wanted others to like me more than anything.

Peta was the only one who could calm me down during my tantrums. She had such a patience when it came to me. She would be still and hug me tight until my hyperventilation ceased.
I would work myself up into such a state.

Yelling, screaming, sobbing, literally losing all emotional control on the floor, and within 15 minutes of her consoling me, I'd settle down. She didn't judge me, and she didn't think I should feel a certain way. Even from a small child, Pete's love and patience had a huge impact on my emotional growth. To her it didn't matter what went down tantrum-wise, in fact most of the time I could barely remember why I was screaming and crying and thrashing about in the first place. Her utter presence significantly transformed my capacity to turn pain into peace. But my self-worth remained low, and if the truth be told,

no one really can save you from yourself.

And so, the battle continued.

There was a history of mental health issues in my family. My great grandmother Greta had suffered chronic depression earlier in her life which saw her hospitalised, and her older brother Art sadly took his own life. My paternal great grandfather George struggled to cope mentally off and on throughout his life and he would seek refuge in nature, opting to live in a cave. My maternal grandfather Ron battled with alcoholism up until his mid-forties. He was a strong and intelligent man, deeply sensitive and creative, and he too battled his own demons. His addiction almost cost him his life, until a spiritual epiphany, as he described it, occurred during a hospital stay in his mid-life and completely 'saved him.' Saved him it did, he never touched another drop, nor did he look back. Pop went on to live the next forty plus years completely alcohol-free, before passing away in his eighties, a fulfilled husband and family man, father to seven, grandfather to fourteen, and great-grandfather to twelve. The struggles of his earlier life had greatly humbled him, and his recovery was nothing short of incredibly inspiring.

Upon honest reflection of my life at 16, I really didn't have a whole lot to be stressed about. I had a great group of friends, I was quite popular, I did well at school, and I had fun. I was your average teenage girl. I experimented with drugs, kissed boys, drank cheap bourbon and paid the price, and then did it all over again. I loved the feeling of escapism. It was a teenage high. And you would think I would have been happy. I mean, I should have been happy. But I wasn't. I was unsettled and I was terribly anxious. It is hard to articulate what was going through my head at the time, but it was like I never really felt grounded, and I couldn't understand why. I was always trapped inside my mind, constantly questioning everything. It was becoming a major problem and everything seemed complicated to me. Yet I was the complicated one.

Complication became clinical depression and I was put on a high dose of medication. Something was definitely wrong, but I didn't know *what* was wrong, and neither did my parents. I was sent off to every therapist imaginable — hypnotherapy, reiki, journey work, counselling, psychologists, and psychiatrists. We tried everything but I just wasn't getting any better. Mum became obsessed with fixing me, but might I say, it was never about getting to the root cause. I knew I was becoming a bit of a problem for her and for everyone. Amongst many contributing factors that kept my mother awake at night, I definitely was one of them. But once again, we didn't talk about it.

Again without a lot of conversation on the subject, I decided to leave school and pursue my ballet. I had been dancing since I was small, in fact movement was in my blood. Mum was a beautiful dancer and she became my first ballet teacher. She opened a little dance school when we were young, intentionally to instil the love of dance in our lives. I loved to dance, although in hindsight I never really gave it my full focus. I held back. Always just a little. Never really feeling like I was good enough to make it. It was the whole 'not walking until I could do it perfectly' thing again. I was certainly very hard on myself.

Going to ballet was familiar and it felt safe. I also wasn't enjoying my strict private school education so the change felt better. It seemed like the right decision to do things differently and so I continued with my studies via distance education. I would finish an entire school term's worth of work within a couple of weeks and spend all day every day at my ballet academy. I absolutely adored my dance teachers, they cared greatly about me and it gave me a sense of value, like I actually belonged to something. There was a sense of community that went with ballet, and a part of me really did love it. But the other part of me was stuck. Stuck in a really low place.

It was the same old story, I felt completely unworthy and out of my depth, and it was all too hard to pursue my goal. I had to find a way out, and find a way out I did. I got a knee injury, which I realise manifested as a way of keeping up my regular pattern. A pattern that perhaps was becoming more of an addiction.

I was addicted to self-sabotage.

I quit ballet and

kissed my dance dreams goodbye,

all the while my psychiatrist prescribed me

the highest possible dose of Zoloft.

At 18 I went to university. When my path to have a career in the arts became a dead-end street, I knew I had to do something. The one thing that my parents had consistently assured me of was my intellect and academic ability. According to them I was always going to be a doctor or a lawyer or a PhD student. There was no middle ground, all I needed to do was focus. So doing what I did best, I instilled the usual ridiculous amounts of pressure upon myself and became the avid over achiever when it came to getting good grades Apparently, I was thriving. Meanwhile in reality, I was getting closer and closer to losing my mind. By this stage I was almost 20, and I lived for the pockets of freedom that a somewhat confused yet normal girl in her late teens would experience. I stayed up all night, I slept all day, and I showed up to a uni lecture every now and then. It was all hard work when it had to be, and then I'd play a hell of a lot harder. Every single week. I was completely self-obsessed, I took zero responsibility, and it felt like the time of my life.

In hindsight I probably was spiralling out of control, but nothing like the out-of-control that would come later.

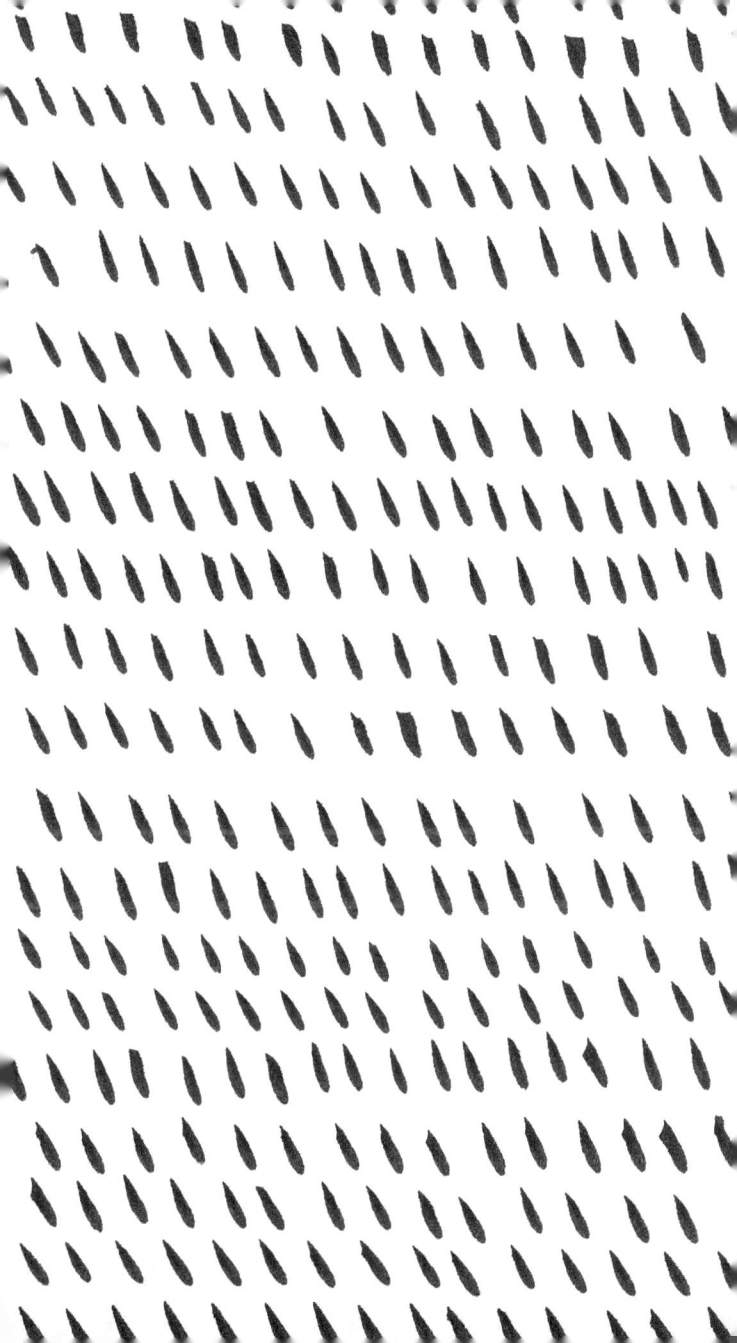

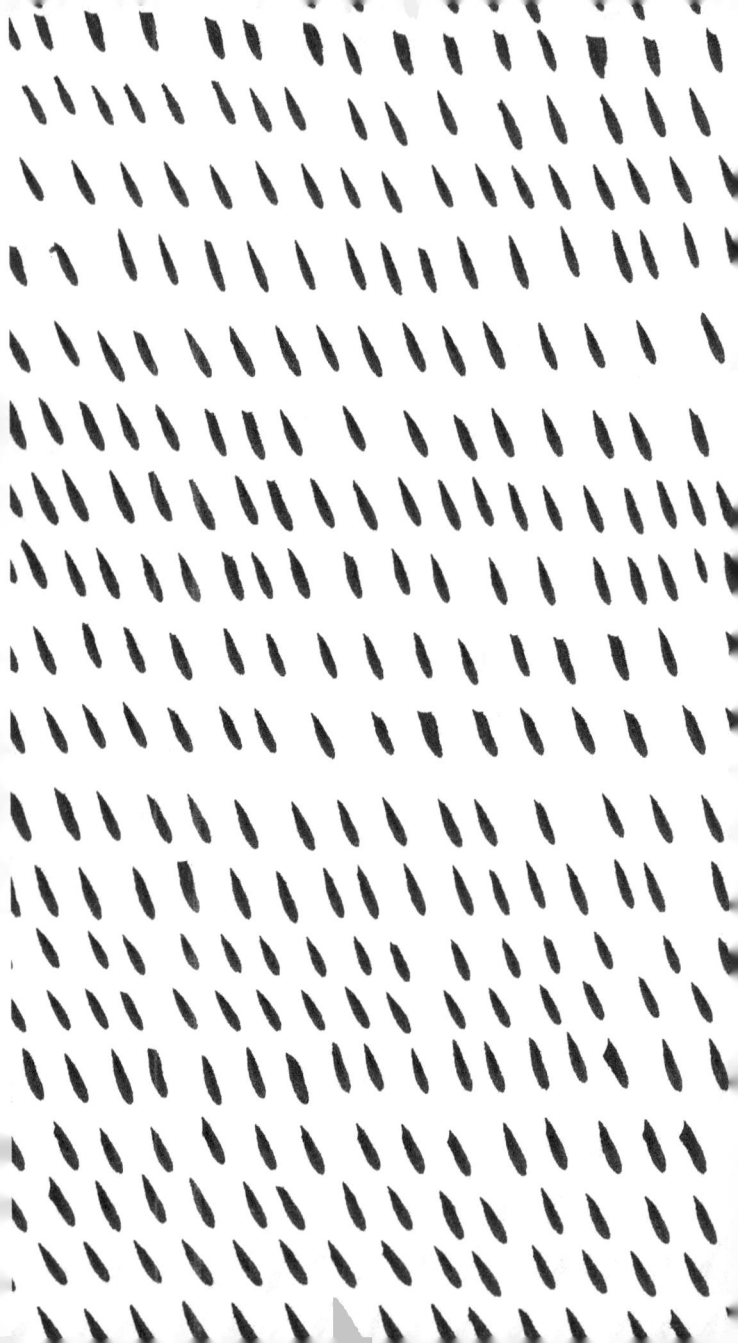

DRIVING ON MARS

CHAPTER TWO

After 29 years of marriage, my parents decided to split up.

As strange as it was, I had always known it would one day happen. I remember as a small child lying awake at night riddled with the fear that our nice little nuclear family would some-day dissolve. I would cry myself to sleep over what was then, nothing other than a figment of my imagination. I never breathed a word of my premonition to anyone, but when it finally did happen, let's just say I wasn't surprised at all.

Personally at the time I was under an abnormally high amount of pressure due to a recent traumatic event, so I didn't have a lot of compassion for either of them. I was frightened and confused and I felt really really alone. I needed my parent's support more than ever before, but they were unavailable. Sure they were going through their own major shit, however I had mine too.

Rather than be supportive, I was angry. Their investment in keeping up the façade of a happy marriage had become way too exhausting for them. I remember the disappointment when it finally did end almost swallowing me up whole. God I blamed them for not sticking it out. Both of them equally. And in my usually-fashioned response to uncomfortable emotions and trauma I distracted myself by working ridiculously hard, and playing even harder. By 'playing hard', I mean sex, drugs and rock & roll, whilst taking zero responsibility for my somewhat reckless behaviour. I felt hurt. I felt let down. And I wanted to blame my parents for being too self-absorbed to notice. I wanted to throw it back at them as hard as I possibly could.

And I found the perfect weapon.

He was unlike anyone I had ever met before.

He had been around the block.

He had the scars to prove it.

And he loved me.

I distinctly remember one particular summer day early in our relationship. The sun was glaring down as we burned our bare feet on the asphalt walking home from the beach. I felt peaceful.

He had his hand in mine, and I calmly said, *"I wish that I could just walk out into the traffic."*

The words escaped my mouth before I could stop them. I felt safe to be completely honest with him.

"Woah," he pulled on my hand to stop me in my tracks and physically manoeuvred me to face him. *"What did you just say?"* He was clearly taken by surprise.

"Yeah," I said in a cool voice, as if I was talking about the weather. *"I kind of dream about walking into traffic fairly regularly."*

Until then, he hadn't realised I was depressed. I remember the look of confusion on his face.

Without judgement, he replied, *"I think we really need to talk about that."*

Meanwhile, my parents discussed a plan to "sort out my depression". The plan was to send me to Canada to work as a nanny and study internationally. It was the perfect solution to get me out of this toxic place. And to be perfectly honest, a combination of my anti-depressant meds, valium, and partying at the time meant that I was really vague and didn't have a lot to say about their grand plan. But the one thing I knew for sure was that no change in scenery was going to fix anything. It had never worked before, so why now would it be any different? *My whole existence* had become a toxic place. *I* was the toxic place. Why couldn't they see that?

With my parents completely absorbed in their own personal struggles, the ground beneath my feet was becoming shakier by the hour. Outside of everyone's awareness, (my own inclusive), things were getting worse. Actually, an atomic bomb was about to explode in my life, destroying everything in its path.

I had my first psychotic episode at a party on the Coast.

I had stopped eating due to a constant churning in my stomach and I think I weighed about 46kg. Mum and dad were away for the long weekend, in a last-ditch attempt to save their marriage. My younger sister Hanna was dancing in Eisteddfods all weekend and I was the one responsible for sewing the last of her costumes.

I was usually good at sewing, but not this time. There I was sitting in front of the sewing machine poised ready to stitch the bright red ribbon trim to her skirt when all of a sudden — I literally could not sew. I was frozen. In an instant it was as if my brain had shut down and I couldn't remember for the life of me how to sew. I had no concept as to how to navigate my way around my very own machine, and one that I'd used time and time again. I still struggle to explain the feeling, it was as if someone had pressed pause on the whole scene and I had absolutely no control over it. The only explanation was that something had definitely changed in my head.

Han was there, watching with this look of incredulity mixed with grave concern. "What is wrong with you? Something is wrong with you" she said reaching over my shoulder and grabbing the fabric I had been fumbling with. "This is not ok. Why can't you just sew it correctly like always? You are not ok", she seemed agitated and confused.

Damn straight it wasn't ok! The costume nor me. In a panic, I phoned mum who reassured me she'd fix the textiles disaster when she returned home the next day. Strangely she wasn't even phased, not for a second, about my sudden inability to sew. I mean clearly it was a common theme at this point in my life to barely have my shit together, but in this instance, it was different. If you can imagine reading your favourite book, and then one day you pick it up and all of a sudden you can't read. As if you've never been able to read. It was terrifying.

Mum did realise I was stressed on the phone that day. Out of concern her response was to encourage me to go to the party that night. "Just go to the party," she said. "Go and have a good time. Stop being so hard on yourself — you don't need to stay at home and sew — a weekend with your friends is exactly what you need."

Reluctantly I took her advice. I picked up my girlfriend on the way and we arrived at the beach house, about 2 o'clock in the afternoon. Typically, it was an hour's drive, and I'd been taking the same route for years so I should've known the way. Strangely, on this day, it took us three hours to get there. I didn't recognise any of the streets; I couldn't navigate. We got lost several times — the universal sign that something wasn't right. I just didn't feel right about the party. And I didn't feel right at all inside my head.

Having built a bit of a reputation for being a party girl, I would normally have felt so comfortable in that kind of environment. On this occasion however, I was particularly anxious and unsettled. I didn't feel I could trust the people around me, most of whom had been my good friends for years. I was amongst a familiar crowd, there were a few strangers, but no one to be concerned about. But still I felt jumpy and unsafe and I struggled to relax.

"Do you want a drag?" The guy sitting to my right leaned towards me reaching out his hand. Instantly the strong herbal smell of the hand-rolled cigarette brought me back to reality.

"Sure", I replied softly. "I'll try anything to calm myself down," I thought but didn't say as I inhaled the joint and passed it on to my friend who was sitting in the darkness to my left. For a moment my mind was still. The continuous barrage of mental chatter had silenced and I remember reclining back in my chair, my attention now focused on the tiny red glow of the lit cigarette as it made its way around the circle.

"Hey Em. Would you like me to get you a drink?" I could just make out his silhouette as he brushed by the back of my chair. My friend was on his way to the fridge and in his usual way was looking out for me.

"Sure," I said. "That'd be great." The party vibe was starting to shift up a gear, a few more people had arrived and someone cranked up the music. But it wasn't just the base that I noticed. Almost in sync with the rise in the volume, so too did the feeling of restlessness rise up from the pit of my stomach.

My friend finally returned with my drink. Surely this would help to calm me down.

"Here's to hoping," I thought as I took a huge gulp of the beer which he had poured into a tall glass. I specifically remember in that instant wondering why the drink wasn't in the bottle? Had the paranoia already set in? I mean, I trusted him, there was absolutely no question of that, but I do recall thinking that drinking from a glass seemed strange.

To this day, I have no certainty as to whether it was the weed or the beer or the slippery slope I was balancing on, but either way, within a matter of minutes, I was completely psychotic.

My brain was completely shattered. Something was desperately wrong and I had no idea as to how to communicate what was going on inside my mind. I will never forget the noise.

In case you're unaware of what psychosis is, it is a condition categorised by hallucinations and delusions in which the sufferer can see, hear, taste, touch and smell things that are in fact not really there in reality. Yet for the person experiencing a psychotic episode, the reality is without question as real as these words are as you're reading them right now. According to Sane Australia; "Psychosis is a mental disorder where a person loses the capacity to tell what's real from what isn't. The causes are complex, genetics, early childhood development, adverse life experiences, drug use and other factors increase your chance of experiencing psychosis. Psychosis requires evidence-based treatment by qualified mental health professionals, it cannot be treated by lifestyle changes and willpower alone."

My head quickly filled up with layers upon layers of loud, contrasting and overbearing white noise. On the inside I was panicked beyond belief, but according to those who were nearby on that fateful night, I appeared nothing other than unusually quiet. Distracted and miles away, consumed in my thoughts.

I can't begin to describe the sheer weight of what it feels like to lose your mind. To begin with, I was able to identify that something had really gone wrong. But my capacity to communicate what was going on inside my head was limited right from the get go. Within minutes, my attempts to ask for help and to articulate my mental state, were drowned out by the noise. Eventually the full-blown craziness would become my reality, as I completely forgot that my previous reality had even existed in the way that it once did.

The layers and layers of sounds and voices remained. There was non-stop screaming inside my head. And then there was the never-ending chatter. I felt like I was channelling everyone's thoughts and conversations like some sort of horror sci-fi film. A completely alternate reality had unravelled and it was all-consuming. There was absolutely no escape.

I desperately wanted to leave the party and I desperately wanted to flee from the noise both inside and outside of my head. Obviously in no state to drive, I reluctantly put myself to bed for the night. There we were, my best friend and I, curled up in a double bed in the guest wing of the house. I lay there staring at the ceiling, bracing for what was to become one of the most traumatic nights of my life. She too lay awake next to me seriously concerned about why all of a sudden I had begun to withdraw and act so strangely. She eventually drifted off to sleep. Me on the other-hand, absolutely no chance. My brain was in next level over drive. I remember being completely obsessed with the idea that people would come into the room and attack us whilst we were sleeping. There was no way I could afford to close one eye let alone two. No one could be trusted. Yet I didn't know why. And the why's didn't matter anymore. The voices continued, all night. They were talking to me. And they were talking about me.

The night seemed to last forever. It was as if I had lived a whole lifetime of torture in my mind before the light of the sun finally broke through the pale blue curtains offering me a second of relief. The bedroom walls were caving in, I literally had cabin fever. With my senses still on high alert, I gritted my teeth and made my way out on to the sand. Perhaps a walk on the beach would bring me back down to earth. But still there was no escaping the noise inside my head.

I was in the grip of a hallucination coupled with crippling paranoia which saw me convinced that every person on the beach that morning was talking about me. Not only could I hear their conversations, but I physically felt their stares of judgment as they passed me by. I couldn't breathe, I was gasping for air. It was as if these random strangers were holding my head under water, and with an evil chuckle they were happy to be witnessing my suffering.

All I could say was, "something is wrong."

I was obsessed with attempting to make sense of it all.

There I was standing, my two feet planted in the cold damp sand, completely traumatised. And insane. And I wasn't the only one who was scared. My girlfriend was now frightened too. Confused and uncertain as to what was happening to me, she just wanted to go home and so did I. Who at that age, or any age, knows what to do or how to deal with a psychotic breakdown?

I drove home, and I swear to God I was driving on Mars.

On the freeway, I continued to hear the conversations of people in their cars as they passed by, and again they were talking about me. As each car passed, I noticed the faces of the drivers were all familiar. They were all people I knew or had known in the past. They were screaming at me from the overtaking lane, "Slut!" "Whore!" "Die Bitch!" Their cars sped past mine with a vengeance as looks of utter disgust blared out from the passing windows. Completely powerless to respond, I did my best to keep the car on the road. I felt like we were traveling at a dangerously high speed. I was absolutely certain we were. A quick glance down at the speedometer and I became even more confused. We were barely moving at 80km per hour.

Powerless to save myself from the paranoid assault inside my mind, there was short-lived relief when I finally pulled the car into my driveway. Still to this day I believe it had to have been divine intervention that got my girlfriend and I home safely that day.

There we stood out the front of my house and for a moment there was total silence. We didn't have a conversation. I just wrapped my skinny arms around her body, breathing in the scent of her hair and holding on as tight as I had been throughout the night. I didn't let go

for a while as I prepared myself for what I knew
lay ahead. I seriously believed that I was going
to die. And it was going to happen soon.
Any minute, any hour, any day now.

I watched my best friend climb into her car.
As she cried, she felt as though I was saying
goodbye forever. And in some ways, I was.

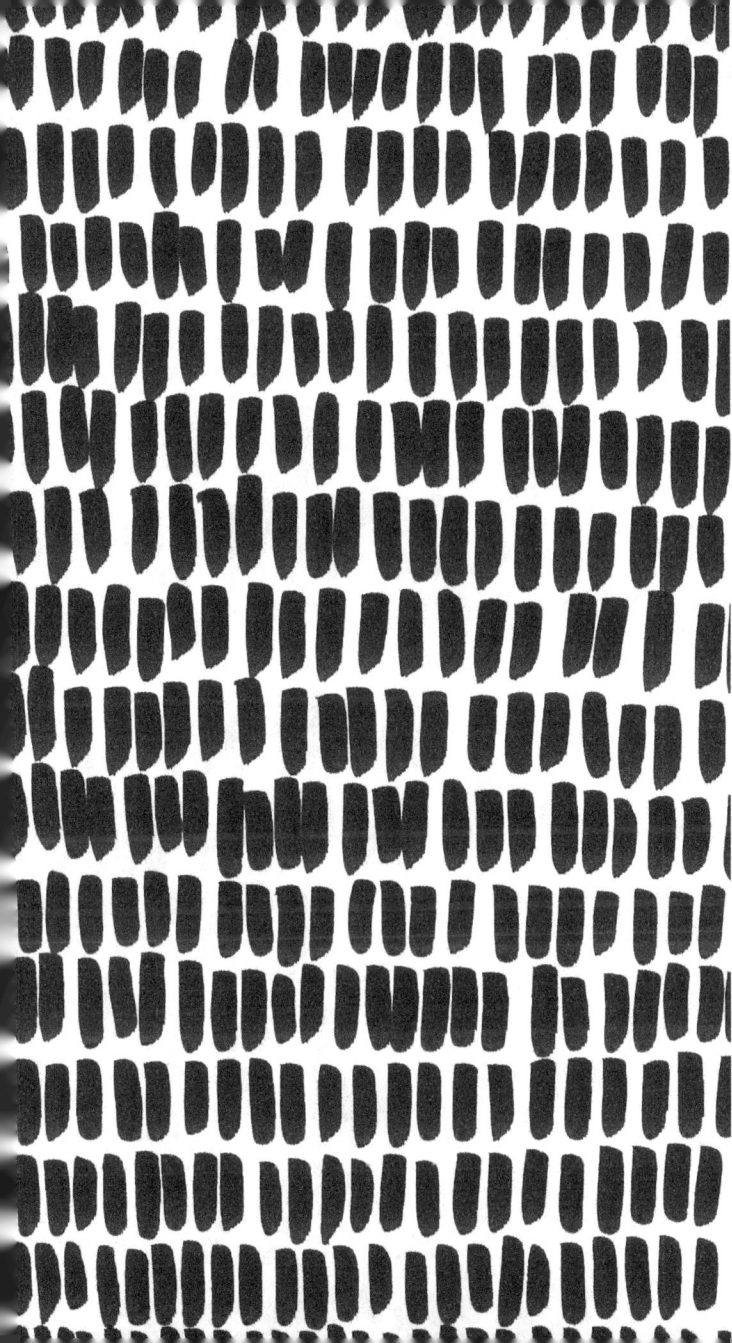

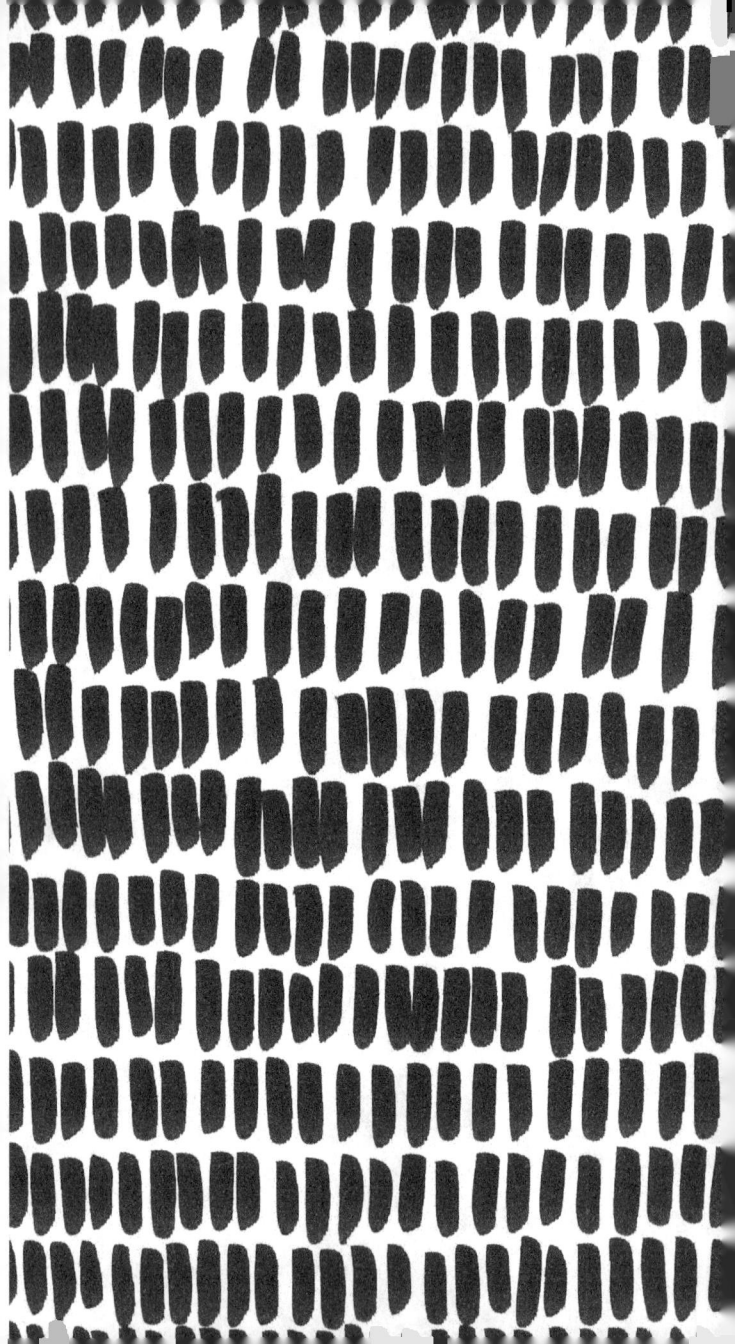

HILARIOUS, TERRIFYING
& COMPLETELY INSANE

CHAPTER THREE

I remember it like it was yesterday. I had walked through a door and there was absolutely no choice to turn back.

After saying goodbye to my girlfriend for what I thought was the final time, I walked into my house and was overcome by an incredible urge to tell my parents that something wasn't right inside my mind. I needed serious help. And I needed them to help me. They had recently returned from their weekend away and were engaged in some sort of informal marriage counselling session involving my uncle and aunt, when I walked into the dining room.

I made a desperate B line toward my mother, and I came straight out with it. "Something is not right with me."

"Hi Emma!" Various voices chimed. I stood there, totally off with the fairies. They were sitting around chatting, holding drinks in their hands and staring at me with half-smiles.

My mum was making her way to the kitchen to check on lunch she had cooking in the oven.

I was hot on her heels, desperate to seek my mother's attention. Now my uncle who is a bit of a joker, had crept up behind me and began randomly putting clothes pegs in my hair. This irritated me.

"Something isn't right!" I raised my voice a little louder. I was frustrated. And I needed mum to hear me.

"What are you talking about Em?" She casually responded as she made her way back to the table to top up the wine.

"I want you to know I haven't taken anything. I haven't taken any drugs." I announced loudly to the entire room. My pupils must've been huge. And clearly, I had zero filter.

"What do you mean?" Dad had a hint of confusion in his voice, having only just joined the conversation, wineglass in hand.

"Well I smoked maybe a quarter of a joint but that's nothing out of the ordinary." I was totally shameless.

My uncle immediately cracked up laughing. They didn't understand; they didn't want to understand. It all seemed to be a bit of a joke to them.

"I think you're just over-tired. How about you go and lie down." Mum stood up from her chair and started shepherding me towards the hallway. She held my upper arm the way nurses lead difficult patients back to their wards. "Emma! You're so incredibly skinny!" She had been away for only three days and I'd probably dropped three more kilos in that time. We stood outside my bedroom door, "You obviously have had a big night. But the main thing is, did you have a good time?" There I was, the voices in my head by this stage screaming bloody blue murder and I felt like I was being dismissed.

I just didn't want to give up. And I had absolutely no idea what was going on inside my head, nor did I know how to explain it to her. So, I gave it one last shot,

"Something's not right."

I repeated again.

"Em, I think you are overtired. You know how you get after a big night. You just need a good night's rest. Off you go to bed." She shut the door. That was it. The pinnacle moment where I could've gone one of two ways.

And the path that I took from then on, I wouldn't wish upon anyone.

So, here's the real corker, which is both hilarious, terrifying and completely *insane* all at the same time: All that I just described from my memories of walking into my house that fateful day, none of it actually happened! It was nothing other than the scenario that played out *inside* my mind! None of it took place on the *outside*. I was totally flabbergasted years later, when my mother told me the real version of events as they unfolded on that same day.

She said that I came home from the party around midday, and she was indeed sitting at the table with my father, aunt and uncle, when I walked in. But I didn't beg them for attention at all nor did I say anything strange or out of line. Instead I walked into the dining room and proceeded to stand there like a total space cadet, a lot quieter and more introspective than usual. My uncle tried to break my distant stare by attaching several clothes pegs to my pony tail. That *did* happen. But even that didn't work to get my attention. I barely even flinched. There was a very brief and uneventful moment of basic small talk, and then completely unannounced, I took myself off to bed for a nap.

It was definitely not some bad dream I could wake up from. And I was accurate in accounting the fact that the noise inside my mind would not ease. I lay on my bed staring at the ceiling in an isolated state of panic; my head wouldn't slow down and I no longer had any handle on reality. Psychosis had become my reality.

I wasn't able to sleep or rest, so upon my mother's actual *real-life* suggestion, in the mid-afternoon of that very same day, I went to Han's dance Eisteddfod. The worst thing was — Mum actually requested that I drive. Oh holy shitballs. Once again, I don't know how we made it there alive. And once again, there I was, out in public, having a full-blown psychotic break.

I know that this will sound strange, but for many reasons over the years, I have wished I could travel back in time to that auditorium on that same afternoon and be a fly on the wall. To be able to observe myself from the outside looking in, namely what I looked like as I unravelled in the grip of psychosis. Symptomatic of the illness itself, I was always unable to see it from any other perspective. I was literally trapped on the set of the horror movie that played on repeat inside my mind. Again, when I asked my mother what this looked like from an outsider's point of view, she remembers me being extremely quiet and wide-eyed that evening as I sat bolt upright in my chair inside the theatre beside her. And on the inside, I was absolutely and totally barking fucking mad.

As I sat there in the audience, my mental plot unravelled. We were being held hostage by a group of terrorists hiding stage-side. Their plan was to kill us all, and they were using the dancers on stage to scene the bloody massacre. The trauma and panic was indescribable. The dancers were wearing white leotards with crosses around their necks, so the religious undertones left me thinking that the bomb was about to go off at any second.

Inside I was tearing my hair out, completely panic stricken but yet there I sat appearing to be completely composed and communicating absolutely none of it to my mother. The more that I watched on, the more panicked I became, I had to do something. Anything. Eventually I worked up the courage to go backstage and find Han. I was beside myself with worry for her safety. I was relieved to find her in the dressing room. I walked straight up to her and took her by the forearms as she stood in her costume fumbling with her pointe shoes. Why was the scene backstage completely unaffected by the threats of violence? Why didn't she realise what was going on? Did she somehow not know that we were all going to die? Of course, she wasn't affected —

No one knew the state of crazy going on inside my mind.

Han was puzzled and beginning to get frustrated by my once again strange behaviour. Thankfully my mother showed up backstage, she took me gently by the hand and guided me back to my seat in the audience.

I don't even remember getting home but I do recall my mother's continuous instructions to go straight to bed and sleep it off. She was put out and confused and who could blame her? There I was, a psychotic, painfully thin ex-dancer myself, acting like a total fruitcake in public and humiliating my sweet younger sister. Seriously.

The sun came up the next day. And nothing had improved.

As I emerged from my bed I realised there was no life on the planet.

It was the dawn post-Armageddon and my two sausage dogs and I were the lone survivors. As totally ridiculous as that sounds, and trust me you can laugh, as I do now, but at the time it was no laughing matter. This was really happening as far as I was concerned.

There was a great silence. A hysterical silence. No longer was there screaming inside my head, but I could hear my heartbeat loud and fast in my ears instead. I knelt down on the floor beside my bed, gripped my dogs, and started to pray out loud for deliverance. *Dear God, please don't*

leave me on this planet alone. I'll do anything,
just please don't forget to take me with you.
Amen.

There was heavy grief in the air. As if I was feeling the depths of a whole world's worth of sadness. I was the only person alive. Everyone had died. It was just me. I was completely alone. Forever. And no amount of praying was going to change this.

As a child, obsessed with the John Marsden series *Tomorrow When the War Began,* I was now living out a scene from the book. A strength arose within me; as if I was a character direct from those pages, I remember thinking: *I will survive this. I will get to the other side.*

In reality, it was a typical Monday morning in my household. I'd slept late and mum was at work, very much alive. Although I don't personally remember this part of the story, apparently I called mum and dad at their respective workplaces and told them they both needed to come home immediately. I told them that I would explain everything once they got home. The *whole* situation.

Mum tells me that her and my father walked into my bedroom, took one look at me sitting on my bed, and knew that it was time to take action. I had sat them down to explain *everything* and in earnest started talking complete and utter gibberish. They couldn't understand a word that I said. It must've been frightening. Straight off to the doctor's we headed.

In my mind I was going to meet with God. The doctor was God. It all made total sense — It was Judgement Day. God would decide my fate, so I had to be on my best behaviour because he was mighty and all-powerful after all. In the meantime whilst I awaited my fate, the doctor's office became a state of purgatory. We were finally summoned in to sit before Him.

"What can I help you with today?" said God, seriously.

"Emma's unwell," said mum. *"She came home from a party a couple of nights ago and wasn't acting like herself and it seems to be getting worse. Her thinking has been affected and something is definitely wrong."*

"I'm fine," I said to God. I needed him to believe that I was fine. It was Judgement Day after all.

"Emma said that she didn't take any drugs at the party but she's definitely unwell," insisted my mum.

"No, I'm not," I said to God. Hands folded in my lap, a serene smile on my pale, drawn face. (*I want to be sent to heaven. Please send me to that better place in the sky*).

"How are you Emma?" God asked me.

"I'm fine." (Act cool, man. Just act cool).

"If the party was more than 48 hours ago, I don't think a blood screening would be useful."

"There's nothing wrong with me," I said. (I am in the presence of God. I am totally at peace).

Meanwhile, mum had risen from her chair and unbeknownst to me she stood behind where I was seated, her arms flailing to get the doctor's attention signalling that I was definitely not okay.

"Look at her eyes,"
she whispered to my God.

"Uh huh, and how long has this been going on?"
questioned God.

"What are you talking about? I'm totally fine."
(If you keep your eyes fixed on God's face and just be super chilled, he will definitely decide you can go to heaven. Just act like everything is normal. Behave and all will be well).

Mum was shaking her head behind me, gesturing wildly to the doctor. He was Indian, and again that made total sense to me. In my head God was definitely Indian.

"How long has this lasted?" asked God.

"We're on day three," said mum worriedly.

"Okay." The doctor knew well and truly that things weren't okay. I was far from fine and he was concerned. He prescribed some more valium and recommended that if my psychosis hadn't eased within 12 hours, a full psychiatric assessment was necessary at the local mental hospital.

I probably should have gone straight from the doctors to the mental hospital that day but my mother didn't want to give up hope. She kept believing that I would wake up soon and be okay. I knew she was praying a lot. She was an avid pray-er.

And there I was thinking all my deluded prayers had paid off. I mean phew. I was just relieved to get out of God's office. I had successfully fooled Him! I couldn't believe it! And although God had decided I wasn't quite ready for heaven just yet, I had been successful in keeping Him out of the hell inside my head. All I needed was a little more time to understand my thoughts and then I'd be more than ready for another crack at Judgement Day.

When I said barking fucking mad. I meant barking fucking mad.

As my attention for a moment wandered off triumphantly, I was blissfully unaware of the actual state my world was in. A state that not even actual sanity could make sense of.

And sadly for everyone, things were going to get a hell of a lot worse.

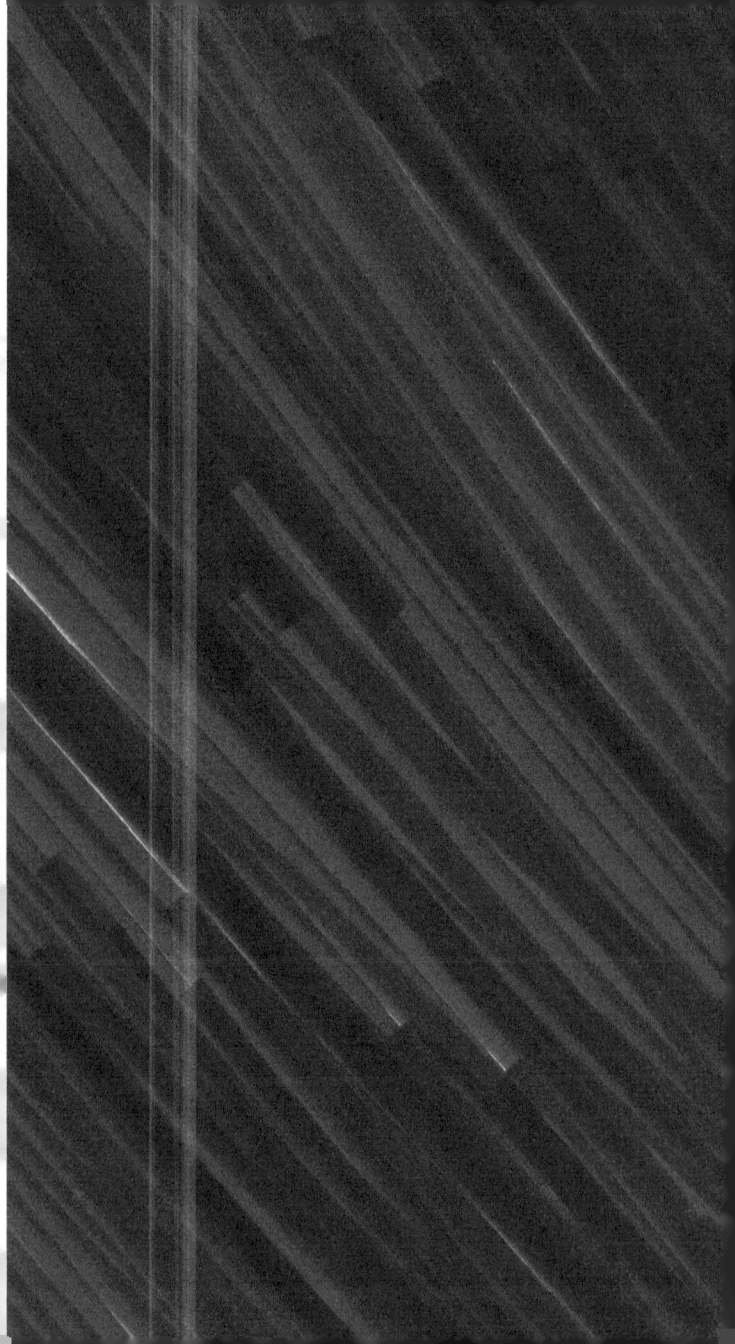

CAN'T YOU SEE I'M BLIND...?

CHAPTER FOUR

Twelve hours later and my mental state had
not changed. Just after dark, I arrived at the
psychiatric hospital admissions centre and
sat between my parents in the waiting room.
Right away the walls began talking to me.
I could hear the souls of people who had been
institutionalised over years gone by. Years of
torment, trauma and frustration experienced by
the clinically insane created layers upon layers
of sound in my mind. I could hear screaming in
my ears, people calling "Help me!", the agitated
were being sedated just two blocks away.

To my parents, it was nothing other than a
boring brick building and a grubby waiting room
not dissimilar to any public waiting area at your
regular hospital. A triage nurse sat behind a
perspex screen staring into her computer, and a
couple of people sat on pea-green plastic chairs
flipping through tattered magazines.

To me it was hell. Just like every movie I had
ever watched set in a psych ward. Strait jackets,
shackles, padded cells, white coats — I could see
it all. This building had a lot to answer for.

Like a young child, I clung onto my mother
and begged her not to leave me there. A nurse

eventually greeted us and took me into an
assessment room where I was met this time
by one of God's disciples — another Indian
doctor — God himself was 'busy'. I was back in
purgatory and again not ready for God or any of
his disciples to decide my fate.

I was no closer to making any sense of the reality
I was living in, I just had to have more time.
I blatantly refused to be admitted.

As an adult in 'the system' I either had to
admit myself into the psychiatric hospital,
or my mother had to commit to taking full
responsibility for my care. The legal term for this
is 'under guardianship,' which deemed me unfit
to make decisions for myself moving forward
regardless of whether or not I was an adult.

It was all up to mum.

If at the time I had been presenting as a danger
to myself or to others, my parents wouldn't have
had a choice in signing me over. I would have
immediately become a Ward of the State.
But luckily, I wasn't there yet. I was acting more
like an infant than a killer.

Neither of my parents felt that this hospital was the right place for their daughter. They certainly couldn't see or hear what I saw and heard, they weren't insane after all. Yet they knew that they simply couldn't leave me there. They had grave fears for my safety inside a place like that.

As a result of their decision I became an out-patient of the Mental Health Crisis Team. For seven weeks I was under 24-hour care. My mother was forced to take leave from work. Various doctors, nurses, care workers, priests, and psychologists were a constant stream through the front door of our family home.

I don't know where to begin in trying to describe what it was like for me. For seven long weeks which felt like a lifetime, I lived in a heightened state of chronic trauma. Every single negative, frightening, or horrific scene I had been witness to previously, on TV, in movies, on the news, or in real life, it *all* became my entire existence. Victimization, isolation, bullying, rape, torture, pain, torment, war, death. You name it, I lived it. I was constantly traumatized and nervous and I was constantly in distress. I couldn't escape it and I couldn't be on my own.

My new reality was as real as the grass is green and the sky is blue. It was as real to me as these words are on the page. I had to physically hold on to somebody, usually my mother, for almost 24 hours a day.

Eventually mum learned that she should stop trying to explain my illness to me. She gave up telling me that I was unwell. I was the child literally stuck in the night terror, and no amount of turning on the light and hugging me saying, "Shhhh, it's not real, you're just having a bad dream," was ever going to help the situation. Whatever you are experiencing, bad dream or not, it is absolutely reality when you're experiencing it — the dream, the nightmare, the psychosis. Your perception. Your reality. Full stop.

The mailman, my sisters, the care workers, the neighbours, the newsreader, my mother... they were all dead. In my mind they had been deceased for weeks now. They looked like zombies, as if they'd been dead for 50 years. Skin rotting away, eyes fallen back in their skulls, teeth and mandible bone exposed — it was complete and utter physical gore, day in and day out. *Total 'Walking Dead' style.*

I'll never forget the afternoon that my mum's best friend called in to offer her moral support.

"How convenient that your name is Di when you're actually dead," I said. I mean she did look like she'd been decomposing for about twenty years. Di appeared well and truly dead to me.

"It is convenient, isn't it!" said Di, completely un-phased. Her capacity to take such confrontation head-on with a sense of humour made her the perfect support for my mum. There they both sat, smiles on their faces as they sipped their mugs of tea. I returned to my silence, staring at Di's grey-green skin, the dark holes where her eyes should've been, the chunks of flesh missing from her arms. My mum's dearest friend was straight from a scene in *Shaun Of The Dead*.

I was afraid of water and wouldn't go into the bathroom without someone there beside me. When it was time to shower mum held me under the running water and I screamed as my flesh melted away under the touch of the acid rain. The shower always rained acid, it was never water. The smell of burning skin infiltrated the bathroom and I couldn't breathe. I was completely traumatised. Eventually when heavily medicated I could sit in a warm bath. I hugged my knees and stared at the tiled walls until someone helped me climb out and towelled me dry.

There were two main underlying themes to my psychosis. It totally polarised. I either wanted to die because everyone else was dead, or people were conspiring to kill me and I was committed to staying alive.

On the days when everyone was conspiring to kill me, it made sense to refuse to take my medication. They were sneaky poison after all. Every time they tried to slip me a pill I would say, "You're trying to kill me again." I was filled with sarcasm. "You still haven't learned...I know your game you do realise." Every move I made was a calculated one. I had to watch my back or else I would die.

I remember one night, sitting around the dinner table. For some reason my father was present on this particular occasion. My brain had a rare moment of realisation.

"Okay, get the camera out — this shit is photo worthy!" My family's forks froze on the way to their mouths as I made them pose for a fake family portrait using a camera I'd fashioned out of thin air with my hands. The home environment was completely broken and we all knew it.

"Check us out all faking it like a happy family, quick get the camera out!" I remember everyone cracked up laughing, slightly hysterical. Because they could see that even through my insanity, I made a lot of sense.

I barely left the house except for the occasional walk around the neighbourhood. Mum had read somewhere that exercise may assist my condition. She'd take me by the hand or let me cling to her jacket sleeve as we strolled slowly through the streets that were once so familiar yet now remained a war zone. Houses were caved in and some had burnt to the ground, cars were smashed and many bombs had gone off. Dead bodies littered the cracked asphalt. The neighbourhood was constantly changing amongst the chaos. The eerie stillness of the aftermath remained. Mum always picked her battles. I never wanted to go for a walk or leave the safety of my home at all, and I usually put up quite the resistance. But on this one day she needed to go out and she had no choice but to take me with her. It happened to be the same morning that I woke up as a blind old man.

"I can't go to the phone shop mum, I've lost all of my vision — I'm blind."

"Emma, come on. Stop it." She rushed around the kitchen and I could hear her jangling her keys in a hurry. She scrunched up some paper and threw it in the bin as her heels clicked on the wooden floor boards.

"I can't come — Can't you see I'm blind!"
My eyes were closed. Literally.

Mum helped me to the car, frustrated and annoyed. "I really haven't got time for this today!"

I point blank refused to open my eyes. I was blind and therefore I needed my mother to help me walk down the street so I didn't fall over or run into things. People were staring at us — it was a fucking scene — a stressed and hurried mother and her stick-thin daughter with eyes closed claiming, "I'm blind, I'm blind." It was like a sad comedy skit.

Her patience was astounding.

She didn't give a shit about what the passer's by may have thought. Mum didn't fear judgement. Nothing mattered to her except my protection.

I didn't think I was pretending. I had my eyes closed, so obviously in real life I couldn't see anything — I felt blind. No one could tell me to open my eyes. It's not as if I woke up and thought, *I'm going to close my eyes and be blind today. What a great idea.* As far as I knew I had suffered a terrible injury and didn't even have eyes to see with. I was blind for the entire duration of the day until I took enough medication to shut me the hell down. Until the next day, when I would wake up as something else, someone else.

My identity changed a lot. I had left my body behind. Throughout the whole of my psychosis I didn't once look in a mirror. There was nothing to see because I didn't exist in the same way. I was completely disassociated for six months at least, before recognising myself as Em once again. The dose of my medication increased over time as it took the doctors months to shut down my episodes of madness. The plot was constantly changing and psychotic episodes lasted 24 hours a day. It was insanity on loop. I would sleep and dream, but then wake up and dream. There was no way of differentiating between sleep and wakefulness. It was a long and complex series of nightmares all rolled into one. My brain never eased off, it never rested.

Day by day I clung to my mother in fear. Her face would often change in front of my eyes. She became the face of a killer, a terrorist, a rapist, a zombie, and I would scream and cry and want for the real her to return. She never gave up on me though. I knew in my psychotic state that even though she was dead, she wasn't going to leave me in hell to suffer alone. She would stay with me until we both could go together to the 'other side.'

"It's mum, Emma," she said attempting to comfort me through her tears. "I'm here. I'm here." She would hold my hand to her ears, watching on as my face was contorted in pain and fear. "Feel mummy's earrings. You know my

gold hoops. Feel them. They're there. It's me.
I'm here."

I touched her face and her hair, but it was
always her jewellery that I recognised as familiar.
The grooves of her gold hoop earrings under
my fingertips brought me comfort and the
knowledge that she was still the real her.

Sometimes I would have moments of apparent
lucidity. When I was calm I loved nothing
more than to tell whoever would listen my
complicated theories and beliefs as to exactly
what was 'going on' and why. My younger
sister Han possibly struggled the most with my
condition, and with what I had become. Han was
in her final years of high school at the time and
was always busy with study and her dancing.
She wasn't home a lot and nor did she want
to be. She didn't have the time to understand
what I was going through, but subconsciously I
think she potentially wouldn't have coped had
she understood my illness anyway. When she
was home it was really stressful for her, and she
found it easier to avoid me. I don't blame Han
at all for her coping mechanisms at the time.
It was beyond confronting. You never knew who
or what was going to come out of me next.
I recall Han often getting frustrated with me and
at times she was flat out embarrassed. It was
stressful and she was frightened. Worst of all
Han was pretty isolated. She really didn't have a
lot of personal support through that time in our

lives. She really didn't know how to explain me to her friends — it was way too full on.

One particular 'mellow' day her and I were lying in my bed together, just chatting. It was almost like the good old days when we were young and life was simple. Her room was next to mine. We lay side by side on top of the covers, looking up at the posters and glow-in-the-dark stickers on the ceiling.

I turned to face her.
"I feel safe to confide in you now."

She rolled onto her left side to look into my eyes, propping her head up on a second pillow.
"Oh really, what do you want to tell me?"

"I'm going to be with you soon," I whispered.

"Huh?" She snorted a quick, confused laugh.

"It's only a matter of time and I'll be with you again soon."

*"But, you're here with me now Em.
What is it that you mean?"*

"No. You think I'm here but you are confused. I'm not really here. I will be soon though, you don't need to worry," I was speaking cryptically.

She didn't know what to say; her mouth moved
slightly as she tried to find words and an
appropriate response, all the while expecting
my resolve to break and for me to crack up
laughing like it was some stupid joke.

I continued, dead serious in my
communication with my little sister.

"I just took the whole bottle of my meds,"

I pulled out the small white empty jar
from under my pillow.

*"All I need to do now is go to sleep, then I'll finally
be with you when I wake up."*

She'd heard enough then.
Han jumped quickly off the bed
and ran to get mum.

I did wake up. The next day, in hospital,
having had my stomach pumped several
times overnight. It's common practice in drug
overdoses for the patient to consume charcoal,
because it binds to the toxic substance and
stops the body absorbing the chemicals. There I
was, drinking black grit through a straw out of
a polystyrene cup for the next few hours.

I remember opening my eyes to an image of the three women in my life, my mother and two sisters, crowding around my pillow peering down at me, their edges blurry. They were all thinking, *Is this finally the end? Is she going to wake up sane? Please may she wake up. SANE.*

Peta used to have a Korean friend named Kit, who would hang out at our house a lot when we were younger, playing in the backyard and braiding my hair and putting on ballet performances in the living room. It had been a long time since we'd all seen Kit.

There was a doctor in the hospital room on the morning I woke up, and she was Korean. She stood by my bedside and quietly asked how I was feeling. The first thing that came out of my mouth when I finally felt I could make reasonable sense of the situation was, "Kit's here. It's so good to see you! I haven't seen you in what seems like forever. What are you even doing here though, did you guys tell her to come and visit?"

I once again had no idea where I was and who I was and who was who. And just like that my family were devastated all over again. I was still clinically insane.

Mum cared for me for four weeks before she had to return to work. By this point, I'd reached a whole new threshold. My episodes largely involved some plot to end my own life.

The mental health team increased my medication again, and the more I was medicated the more I slept. My brain needed to shut down to give it the best chance to repair. From how it's been described to me since, it was as if an atomic bomb had erupted inside my brain and all the neurons were in complete disarray. Which meant none of my thinking made sense, nor did my emotions. My head was one big jumbled mess, which meant pretty much the same for my perception of reality. I could hear, see, touch and smell things that weren't in fact *real*.

But after all, perception really is in the eye of the beholder, and it was one hell of a crazy reality in which I was living.

People with chronic psychosis typically get hospitalised as they are unable to care for themselves. Fortunately, I had my immediate family, and I wasn't showing any signs of putting anybody else's life at risk, nor was I violent, which is a common myth when it comes to psychosis. For a long time, society has believed that people who are suffering psychosis have an increased likelihood of violence, but this isn't actually true.

Regardless of the facts though, in accordance with my hallucinations I believed that everybody else was already dead, therefore no further harm could really be inflicted.

Being the only person on the planet alive, I really was the only one in harm's way.

Subsequently my mother decided that
the whole house had to be Emma-proofed;
chemicals, knives, scissors, razors, anything
sharp was hidden out of my reach. I'd also for
some strange reason developed an overnight
obsession with cutting my own hair. I distinctly
remember this one particular day when mum
had to work. A very brave girlfriend had stepped
in to care for me. She had taken me for a drive
and out of nowhere I began attempting to throw
the contents of my handbag out the car window.
In my mind — why need a handbag? I was the
only person on the planted alive remember.
So there was no need for wallets or makeup.

Peta moved back home temporarily to help take
care of me after mum had to return to full time
work. Having her around worked wonders.
We'd always been incredibly close. I trusted her.
She knew what I needed almost intuitively.
We'd walk along the foreshore whilst watching
the waves rolling in and out near the lighthouse.
She'd hold my fragile hand and we'd breathe in
the fresh salty air. It was peaceful.

Then all of a sudden, her legs
would be blown off.

This one time, I sat bolt upright in the middle of
the night riddled with panic, grief and guilt that
I hadn't been there to protect Pete from the blast.
She had been involved in a car-bombing planted

by the enemy. In my ability to see the future, I knew that the bomb was there under her car. I could have saved her, I could have saved her legs. I ran down the hallway from mum's room tears streaming down my face and carefully peered around the doorway to her bedroom. I was frightened of what I would see but I had to look despite my fear. There she was, sleeping under the blankets. Her flame-red hair spread out on the pillow confirmed the truth: you see she'd also been burnt in the attack, and her hair usually dark brown, had adapted to the colour of the fire.

I ran into the room, launched at the bed and wrenched the blankets off her sleeping body. Devastated to see the little stumps that were once her legs. Pete woke with a start to see me clutching at her legs as I descended into utter sympathy and deep sadness for her loss. The best thing about my older sister was that rather than telling me that she did in fact have her legs and it was all just another episode in my crazy head, she went along with it. When my panic became sadness she understood that maintaining my sense of calm was most important for my mental health. She looked at me lovingly and explained how there was no need to be sorry. She could still walk and move despite having little stumps for legs. She would now get around on a skateboard. I had such a sense of relief that despite losing her legs, she was going to survive.

On my quest to always make sense of the craziness, one day I decided I finally had it all figured out. Again. I knew exactly why this was happening to me. I finally knew perfectly and clearly what was going on.

This time I knew I was on the money.
I couldn't wait to explain it.

"Pete, we need to go outside," I whispered, with eyes wide and a huge grin spreading across my face. We were curled up together on the couch, my head in her lap as she watched the news. It was another rare moment of lucidity. I had been silent for at least an hour.

"Ok, why?" She began to question.

"Let's go outside. I know. I mean I really know what's going on. Come with me and I'll explain." Despite my excitement, I spoke with a hushed voice, because *the people* were always watching and listening.

Peta followed me to the front yard. My eyes shone with clarity. For a moment she fully believed I'd had a real breakthrough and she was committed to whatever I was going to say or do.

It was early in the evening and I stood by the

front fence preparing for my sermon. My sister waited with bated breath, her heart pounding.

"Look up at the stars." I gestured, reaching my arms to the sky. *"We really all are just a tiny blip in this massive universe. And I know now exactly what I am and exactly who I am. Everything that I am going through, it all makes entire sense. I can't believe it took me this long to figure it out, but better late than never, that's for sure"* I spoke with clarity.

"Really? Wow!"
Peta was enthralled by what I was saying, but me acting like some high priestess all of a sudden had planted the seeds of doubt in her mind. My state of crazy was slowly becoming apparent again.

"I'm a worm," I announced.

"What?" Her brow furrowed slightly, but she knew she had to go along with it.

"I've had it wrong for a while but I've finally got it now. I'm not a human. I'm actually a worm."

"Ok, Em. Tell me what you mean." A small, encouraging smile painted across on her lips.

"I'm a worm. I mean, I'm a strain of virus."

"Why?" Pete asked.

"Because they can survive anything,

and I'm not dead yet.

So that's what I have to be.

I'm a worm.

A kind of bacteria.

They can't kill me."

Once again everyone else in the entire world
including her was dead. I was the only one left,
so I had to have been a worm — it's the only
thing that made total logical sense.
Right? God. Help. Me.

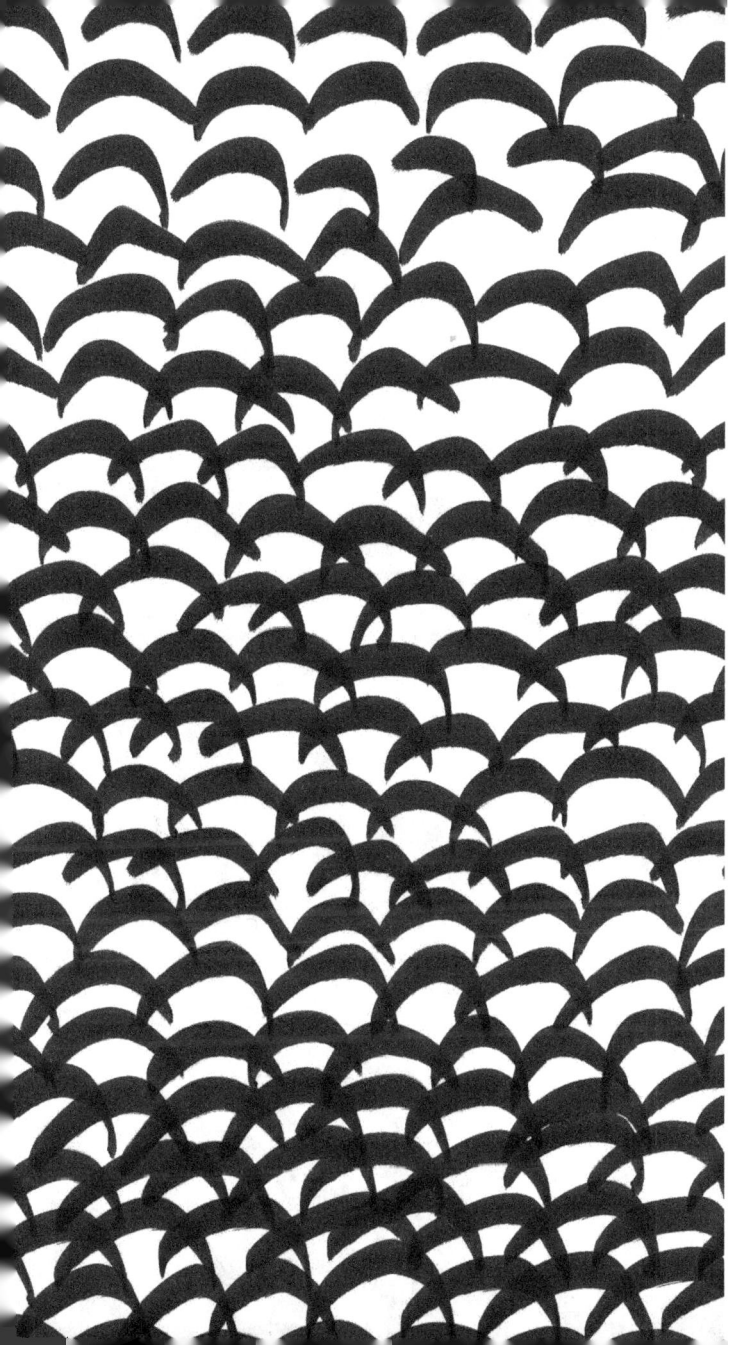

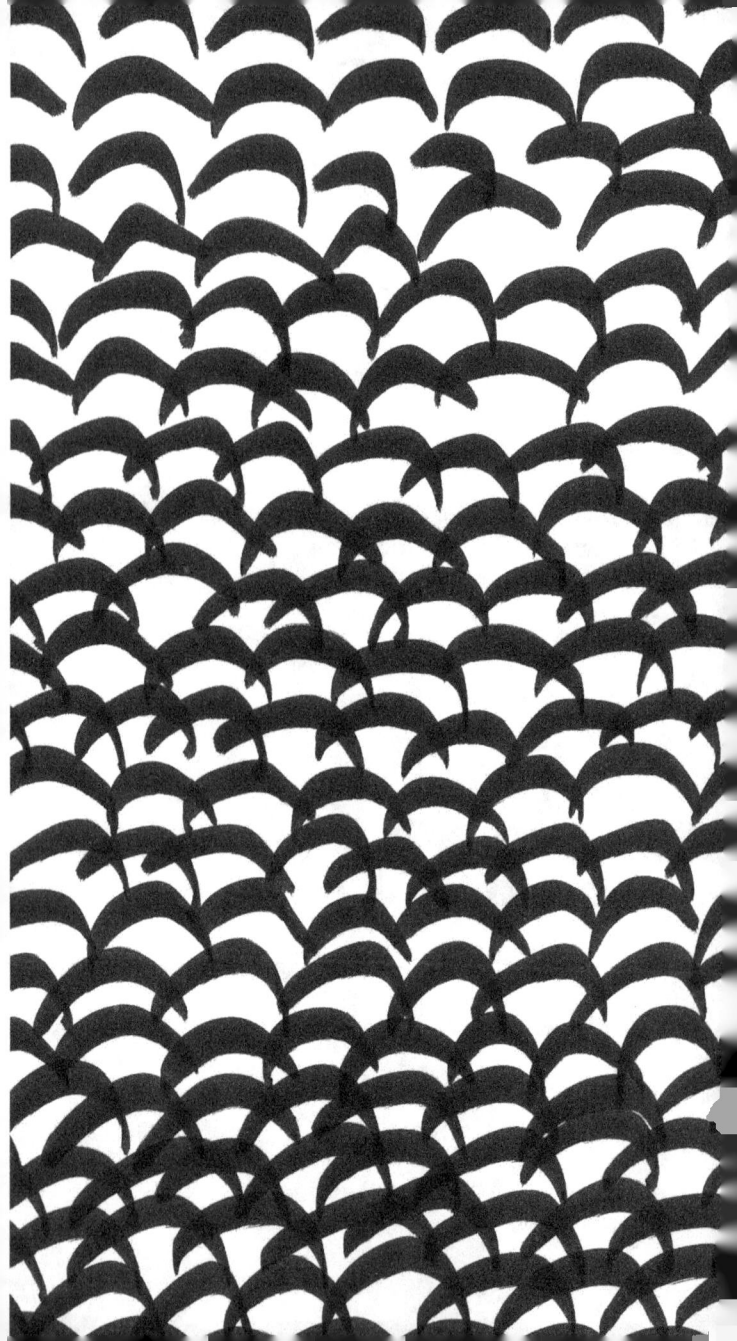

THE CRISIS

CHAPTER FIVE

It was beyond difficult. Not just hard for me,
but hard for everybody.

It's a universal fact that nothing can compare
to a mother's love, but it never really rang true
for me until I became a mother myself. When I
was insane my mother's commitment to me was
unshakeable. I trusted her, I leaned on her, and
it changed our relationship forever. As a small
child you will recall I clung to her like a life raft.
During my teenage years it got complicated
and we drifted apart as mothers and daughters
often do whilst navigating the challenges of
adolescence. I chose to rebel rather than to
listen to her. We were both on our own separate
journeys. Then came my illness, and I was like that
small child again.

It was difficult to get an accurate medical
diagnosis. In most cases psychosis is
experienced as an episode where the symptoms
are acute. But as my symptoms became chronic,
whereby my reality day in and day out became
one prolonged hallucination, the medical
practitioners responsible for my treatment
believed that the psychosis was occurring
as the result of another mental illness. Was

it schizophrenia, schizoaffective disorder or bipolar? It was a case of treating me for the worst and hoping for the best, but either way the prognosis didn't look good and my family were devastated.

My mother dropped everything and could do nothing but be my carer. It was all about fighting for my survival. As time went on and my illness progressed, she started to realise the truth; that I might never get better. It honestly looked like she would become the long-term guardian of a mental patient. Despite her commitment to my care, there was a part of her that never truly accepted I would be ill forever. A small part of her believed in miracles, believed that I would one day be her Emma again. The little girl that she cherished stayed in the forefront of her mind and she fought hard for me to get better in any way possible.

I can't even begin to imagine what it was like for her during those years enduring her own pain amidst a marriage breakdown as well as caring full-time for her middle child who had become a semblance of her former self. My illness served as a dramatic wake-up call for her. Instead of simply *doing* motherhood, she was forced to *be* a mother. It's all she could be during that traumatic time. Caring for somebody physically sick is difficult, but caring for somebody who is severely mentally ill is a whole other level. And she was largely on her own at that time with no great support network or resources. My father was often absent, on the road for his career and going through his own personal struggles. Not being around much meant that he didn't have the capacity to fully understand my situation or hers. At the time she really took it all in her stride though, she felt she didn't have a choice. She had to be strong. She was fiercely protective and wanted to remain in control of my care, the way a new mother hovers over the shoulder of a new father while he bathes their baby for the first time.

In some ways I believe my illness offered mum a distraction from her own problems; her focus became about keeping me alive. She put her own needs on the backburner for a time. Whether that was good or bad it didn't matter, because I required such a high level of care and attention — There simply was no other option. Mum didn't see any other way but to power up and keep going no matter how tough it got.

The life we all knew was crumbling around us yet it seemed to make her more patient. There was a lot of shame surrounding my illness but mum never made it known that it affected her.

I was still just her little girl. People still to this day do not have a great understanding of severe mental illness, or what it was like at that time under our roof.

If you can imagine for a moment a house with a daughter like something out of *The Exorcist?* Then yes, you'd be right in assuming not many people wanted to visit.

I labelled myself "The Crisis,"

as it was the Mental Health Crisis Team that were regularly doing in home visits to check up on me. It was a name that made total sense to me at the time, and funnily enough it stuck. Still to this day there's a running joke in our family that I take the cake for being the craziest person anyone could have ever met at that time. Yet through the laughter and sometimes hysteria surrounding my past, they also consider me to be the sanest person they know now. I went from the depths of insanity to resurface and become more sane than ever before. And there was no miracle nor mystery behind how I did it. But more on that later.

Whilst the power of a good sense of humour should never be underestimated, mum still can get emotional when we talk about the past. My illness impacted her life dramatically and she carries the trauma somewhere far back in her mind the way most mothers would. Only recently she told me a story I hadn't heard before, or perhaps it was one that I'd blocked out. Among the many changes I went through as a psychiatric patient, one of the biggest changes I grappled with was the fact that I physically looked different. I had put on more than 25kg. Weight gain is a common side effect of anti-psychotic meds and I was on a high dose to manage my condition which resulted in a very slow metabolic rate. I slept all of the time and was ravenously hungry when I was awake.

It was a random Saturday afternoon at home in the lounge room. I was sitting on the sofa in front of the TV eating some variety of fast food. Peta was visiting from the city and she was overcome with emotion at seeing me sitting there in a medication-induced haze consuming junk food, all swollen and vague and barely recognisable. I was not the same person mentally nor physically and Pete was really struggling to cope with the dramatic change.

"Look at you." she cried, storming right up to me snatching the food right out of my hands. "What is wrong with you?! Who are you?!!!! I just want my sister back! I want my Emma back!" She screamed at me in frustration.

Mum rushed into the lounge room at the noise. Her heart broke to see me sitting motionless on the couch, tears pouring down my face with utter confusion and helplessness as Peta cried and yelled. My sister missed me, deeply. She missed our friendship, she missed who I used to be, and she was struggling to accept that I would live out the rest of my life like this. Of course mum understood her pain because part of her feared the same. They really were locked in shock and grief at the sudden loss of who I once had been. But to my mother, she was just grateful that I was alive and no matter what — I would always be her little girl.

Mum's biggest fear for me was that she genuinely couldn't protect me from the outside world. If she couldn't protect me from the frustrated attack fired by my own sister, how could she ever protect me against the rest?

She felt like she was powerless to save me from the misunderstanding and stigma surrounding severe mental illness,

psychotic breakdown, and what had become of me. She worried deeply for the life I had ahead of me, full of judgement, shame and humiliation. It was the kind of despair and overwhelm of emotions that she had never experienced before.

Or perhaps she had experienced it before? Perhaps that was why she seemed to be a master at coping. Or was she just a well seasoned expert at masking stress? One thing I learned quickly about my mother from a young age was that she certainly had perfected the art of keeping her feelings to herself. Bearing the depths of her emotions made her vulnerable, and this was something she certainly was not comfortable with. A deeply private person, sometimes as if she was coated in steel. Yet when others outside of herself are in serious darkness she cracks right open and rises up, drawing upon a faith and love that is deeper than the ocean. The woman is selflessness incarnate.

Besides my illness mum had been through a hell of a lot over the years and there was so much that I really didn't understand. I yearned to know her story, as I did my father's. Grasping where they came from in more ways than one was only going to help me better understand myself. To close doors. To open others. To forgive. To heal.

My father had a fairly regular run-of-the-mill childhood. Growing up in the country as the youngest of three boys, he got to experience a real sense of freedom that was playing outdoors among green rolling hills, trapping rabbits, climbing trees and swimming in the icy cold water of the creek that ran through his family property. During Christmas holidays he travelled to the city to stay with his grandparents whilst seaside holidays recurred regularly on the annual calendar for the family to unwind. His father was a school teacher which meant they moved around to meet his work requirements all while dad's mother took great care of the home.

My dad was a high achiever for as long as he could remember, he respected authority and loved his parents greatly whilst never wanting to let them down in any way. Having learned this about him, I quickly drew a parallel to the people-pleasing-self I often grappled with. Perhaps I had adopted this behaviour from him? In his own career dad reflected the strong and influential values his parents possessed. My grandfather's motto in life was "knowledge maketh man," which instilled a belief in my dad that education and learning was a vital key to a successful life. His mother taught him, through continuous demonstration, the art of unconditional love whilst insisting on the importance of self-belief and "going after your dreams." She was a striking and faith-filled woman, and one incredibly wise human being. "Granny", as we called her, had a presence and grace about her that impacted many lives significantly, mine included. She was famous amongst family and friends for her quick wit and hilarious one liners. There was one particular joke that stuck in more ways than one — the use of her self-created word concept coined 'fith.'

F.I.T.H. was an acronym which stood for 'Fucked In The Head,'

and one could suffer from a case of 'fith' mildly or severely dependent of course upon the circumstances surrounding the said case. A slight error in judgment could be classified as a fleeting moment of 'fith' in her book, where as a more significant mistake, perhaps leading to some kind of drastic life change, could be pegged down as a more severe case. *One might say I had fith at the more severe end of the spectrum. As much as granny was never serious, this little joke taught me a great deal about the need for compassion when it comes to human error. People do make mistakes and we do fail, but screwing up is central to the human experience, central to living, for without our mild cases of 'fith' how do we ever get to learn and grow and become who we are here to become?

Unfortunately for me, my severe case of 'fith' became no joke. There was nothing funny about it. But by god did the lessons remain.

Together with my sisters we absolutely adored our paternal grandmother. She was more than our granny, she was a soul mate. I only wished I could have had more time on this earth with her, and I know my father feels exactly the same way.

Dad struggled greatly with complicated grief after his mother's passing and sadly he didn't seek the professional help he deserved and greatly needed. Whilst navigating his way through the loss, grief and his own 'fith' meant that he began making choices that would affect the course of his life in a way he could never have predicted.

And one choice he would make eight years after my grandmother's death, would change my whole world forever.

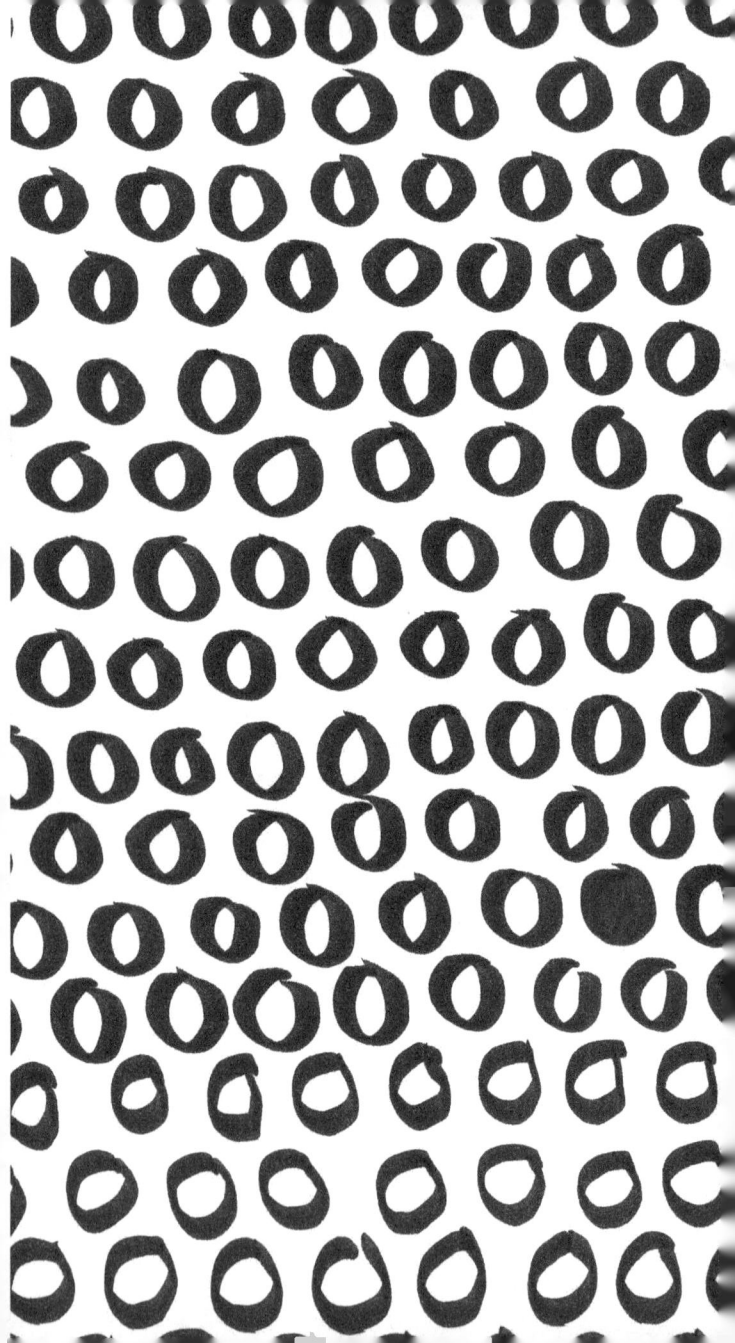

SLIM SHADY

CHAPTER SIX

My father had been taking care of me for
only a few hours before he took me to the
mental hospital.

After seven weeks, mum and Peta had to go
back to work and I still required round-the-clock
care. Up until this point not much had changed
for dad as he worked away a lot of the time.
He was also fighting his own demons, which
left very little room for mine.

Strangely during my psychosis, I was terrified of
my father. I guess because he wasn't around a
lot. During my episodes he wasn't who I thought
he was, he was other people, bad people,
people I didn't trust. The day I finally became
a Ward of the State, I sensed within minutes
that my father was ill-equipped and put out by
having to look after me.

"How are you Em? How are you today? How is
she today?" He asked questions without waiting
for the answer, talking over the top of my head
to my mother as she hurried out the door to
get to work on time. I wouldn't speak to him.
He pulled his phone from his pocket and went
into the kitchen to make a cup of coffee.

In the pit of my stomach, I knew the day was not going to go well. My mind told me that I couldn't trust him. He was on the 'other team' and now he was here, in my safety zone at home, and my one and only protector — my mother — was gone. I peered around the door frame from my bedroom, watching his every movement thinking cryptically, "Just do what you came here to do. I'll say nothing. Simply get it done. Or leave."

I recall waking up from a deep sleep and I had wet the bed. The linen was a mess and dad had no time for it. I remember he was unsympathetic and frustrated as he removed the sodden sheets from my bed and threw them in a pile on the floor.

"What is wrong with you?" He gritted his teeth and stared in my direction.

I don't know if he actually spoke to me, or if it was all in my head, but I certainly felt like he was questioning all that was wrong with me. Ashamed and humiliated, I offered him no response. His phone rang and broke the silence. He stormed out to the back courtyard, holding the mobile phone to his ear and pacing back and forth. I knew I had just become another huge problem for him.

I watched him for a minute or so, through the glass doors leading outside, then I proceeded to lock myself in the bathroom. *Screw this, I'm out of here and out of you.*

At the back of the cabinet, I found disposable razors. The only sharp objects that hadn't yet been hidden from me. I filled the bath and desperately hacked at my wrists, attempting to do enough damage that would take away the pain. I submerged my entire body fully clothed in the warm water. *I'll just die. It'll be sweet. Let's just get this over with.* It was as if I thought by taking control of the situation, he couldn't get to me. I was sick of feeling like I had to explain myself to him. To everyone. I knew that no one was going to save me, and certainly not him, so I just had to die. Everything would be fine once the madness had ended. *Please make it end.*

Dad was banging on the locked bathroom door, shouting at me to open up, to let him in. I could feel his panic and fear on the other side of the door. That was definitely real. But I didn't let it affect me and my decision. *Soon the hell will be over.*

He called the Mental Health Crisis Team and they arrived quickly, because I was on high alert.

I *was* the Crisis after all. On some level, I knew that they'd arrive, and perhaps I thought they could rescue me from the shame I felt around my father.

A team of four mental health workers broke through the bathroom door. I remember one male nurse scooping me out of the bath, and there I stood on the tiles weak and exhausted, sopping wet and fully clothed as they wrapped me in towels. My father sat beside me in the back of their van, tears streaming down his face. I was stoic. Relieved to soon be free of his judgement.

We arrived in the admissions area of the mental hospital and the screaming began. The walls were talking again. I could hear it all and feel it all, but on this particular day I didn't let it get to me. I didn't care anymore. I was going in, no matter what.

"Are you sure you want to be admitted?" Dad asked me, clutching my bandaged wrist, his eyes filled with tears. The lady behind the counter was a grey blur. I refused to look him in the eye. I just wanted him gone.

"Yes." I responded calmly. It was only going to be a matter of time before mum would come and recuse me. I was certain that as soon as she finished work she'd be there to take me home giving me no reason to stress.

A nurse took me through to my dorm and dad followed. A white room with four single beds. She led me to the bed closest to the door and I curled my tiny frame in a cross-legged position on top of the sheets. I remember watching the clock, counting down the minutes until mum would finish work. It was just after noon.

"Do you want me to go?" Dad asked.
He looked frightened.

"Yes, I want you to go. There's no need for you to stay. Mum will be here soon." I replied softly,
still refusing to make eye contact.

I watched him through the large perspex window, overcome with emotion and struggling to make his way back to the main entrance. His little girl was now a Ward of the State, and he immediately felt the weight of that decision. I, however, was none the wiser.

**That's when the woman threw
the book at my head.**

At the time, I didn't recognise I was in a mental hospital, or who the scary lady was rocking back and forth on her bed. I had no idea that there were many terribly ill people in this place, all like me, all insane in some way or another. All I knew was that wherever I was, I needed to be here so that my mother could return and finally remove me from the care of my father. This place? This place was temporary. She'd be here soon.

My ward wasn't the ward where the killers go — you know, the people who plead insanity in court and take asylum in mental hospitals. They were still there though, among us. We all had yard time together. Far out, there were some sights to see in that place. It sounds like prison, doesn't it? Well, believe me, it wasn't far from it. We were all kind of stuck in there together.

There was no lock on the door of my dorm room and my family had grave concerns for my welfare. You see there weren't many other 20-year-old girls weighing 40-something kilos inside that place. Mum and Pete were constantly fearing for my life, particularly when I didn't have the capacity to understand what real life even looked like. They were forced to fight really hard to make sure I received a certain level of care. I was so fortunate to them as many of the people inside those walls had no one to fight for them.

As my level of sanity gradually improved while in hospital, the more I began to recognise my existence. And the more horrid my real-life situation became. I felt groggy, dazed and confused as I slowly woke up from the nightmare, only to find my new reality just as traumatic.

It was a rollercoaster that lasted months and months. Prolonged weeks with round-the-clock care at home: one long episode of trauma that never ceased. Now surrounded by a whole bunch of other crazies in an asylum. It was next level madness.

I remember on the day I was admitted I was gently coaxed off my stark white single bed to join my new friends for lunch at the cafeteria (to this day, food halls make me very uneasy). I still wasn't eating much at that point because I was yet to give up my belief that food was poison. The smell in the cafeteria was disgusting, and I don't know if that was real or the psychosis, but there was no way I was eating any of it. I remained painfully thin for those first few weeks.

One time boobs were served up for lunch. Yeah, you read that right. Mum was visiting me, so it must have been a weekend. I picked up my grey plastic tray from a pile near the door, and shuffled slowly along the line as faceless bodies spooned apparently edible piles of colourless slop onto our chipped and grubby plates. Pop music blared through a tiny speaker in one corner of the hall, slightly drowned out amid the sounds of clanging pots and pans in the adjacent kitchen, murmured chatting at the tables, people barking, occasional screaming. The usual madness.

Mum and I sat at an empty table near the door. She pulled a tissue out of her purse and began wiping up the remains of someone else's lunch.

"What the hell is this?" I was shocked.

"Sorry... what, darling?" Mum quickly pulled another tissue out of the packet in her bag, ready to attend to any remaining oily mess on the table surface.

"What are you doing trying to serve me boobs?"

Her brow furrowed slightly: an effect I had on many people during my crazy days. Everyone had a visible moment of confusion, during which they debated how to react, whether I was joking, should they ignore me, placate me, laugh, or go along with it? It must have been stressful and exhausting to say the least.

"Boobs!" I screamed. *"Fucking boobs!"*

I was staring down at my plate in disgust. A vision of two perfectly round and perky boobs, nipples standing to attention, sliced right off and arranged in alignment on the plate in front of me.

On this occasion, my mother cracked up laughing. She attempted to calm me down — I was screaming and carrying on — but laughed all the while. How could you not?

I pushed my tray aside and, just like every other day, refused to eat the body parts on my plate. Where on earth did I get that from? I haven't seen that many horror movies, I swear. It was horrid. A traumatic nightmare. And kind of hilarious. What had become the story of my life.

I entered hospital fairly unstable given that I didn't even know where I was at the time. It took about a month for me to stabilise, wake up and gain some level of understanding as to where I was and how the hell I got there. It was incredibly traumatic for my family to see me in this dingy place, but they all did an amazing job at hiding their fear from me. I was constantly supervised by the nursing staff so I couldn't hurt myself or others, but besides that, there wasn't a real lot to do in there. It was incredibly eye-opening and confronting for my family to see mentally ill people in this environment, removed from society and any sense of a normal existence, trapped inside their suffering minds. Who ever thought I would end up right there with them?

At one point Peta advocated hard to have me moved into a different room because my ward was really filthy and run down and it just didn't feel safe in her opinion. I was moved after a few days of her making the complaint and the next weekend she visited my new room. While opening all the drawers and checking the cupboards, she found a large bottle of bleach right there in broad daylight in the bottom of the closet. The door wasn't locked, which meant any patient could get at it. Just imagine, a full bottle of bleach in the hands of psychotic people. She absolutely lost it as any sane responsible person would.

My family can still get upset when we talk about my time 'inside' (which isn't often), and about the system that fails so many. It was hard for them to witness my level of care, or lack thereof, not to mention the other patients who had no one to even visit them. I now realise that it's a serious public health concern, greatly worthy of more resources and attention. Cue the fire in my belly just thinking about the possibility of creating change for the better in this space.

I remember seeing a lot of tortured faces in that hospital. And a lot of nudity. I had a really good sense that I wasn't in Kansas anymore that's for sure. The people around me were foreign, and not friends. I was definitely frightened a lot, but I was more subdued now, no longer on high alert in the way that I was at home. I met a lot of different patients and I heard a lot of different stories.

At one point, I shared a room with a mother of three young children who was undergoing electric shock therapy for chronic depression, a treatment method I didn't even realise still existed. I mean we had entered the 21st century and there I was thinking that shock treatment was from back in the dark ages. Silly me. I met a man with a massive indentation in his skull, just looking at his head scared the bejezus out of me. He had been in such a severe motor accident that he never recovered from the post-traumatic shock. There were anorexics, drug addicts, schizophrenics, and criminals.

Suicide attempts were common, violence often erupted, sedation pills and tranquilliser injections were regularly prescribed. Insanity at its worst, and all in the one place. It was a horrific place to be. I honestly struggle to find the words for it. And among it all, the sound of the constant, constant screaming.

The real Slim Shady was in hospital with me.

He was a highlight. Well, he thought he was. In his opinion he was dead set Eminem: he wore the same outfit from the original album. White singlet, denim shorts, headscarf. He walked like Eminem and called himself Slim. It was a crack-up because he clearly thought he was the real deal. Most of us probably did too. At that time, it was impossible to know what was real and what wasn't.

Was this dude a figment of my imagination?
Or was the real Slim Shady actually standing up
right in front of me? It was all very confusing.

Slim took a fancy to me; he followed me around.
"Got a ciggie bruz?"

One night, I woke up and he was sitting on
the end of my bed. *"Got a ciggie bruz?"*
That's all he ever used to say on repeat.

I woke up in my pink flannelette pyjamas and
there's Slim perched somewhere near my right
knee. I kind of liked him, he was harmless,
but still it was getting close to midnight.

"No, I don't have a ciggie."
I replied sheepishly, hoping he would go away
without a fight. He wandered off in the darkness
on his quest to find a smoke.

No one else was around that night and it was
lucky all he wanted was a cigarette because
I wouldn't have stood a chance. That was
the reality of life in there. Even if I were to be
attacked, or if any of us were for that matter,
who could we tell? And would they believe us?
The claim could always be "she's making it up",

"she's mentally ill." This in itself was a very confronting reality.

Meanwhile, the medication was shutting down different parts of my brain so that it could begin to heal. I moved from a state of trying to consistently make sense of my thoughts, to actually not even having the capacity to reason or make sense of them at all. I slept for long periods, sometimes up to 18 hours per day.

I'll never forget the time we watched *Love Actually* during one of the ward 'in-cursions'. Once a month or so the nurses would clear a large area in the common room and line up the hard-plastic chairs right in front of a pull-down projector screen. We all filed into this makeshift cinema, none of us having a clue what the hell we were doing there all sitting in a row. It was like the scene of some black comedy show before the opening credits had even rolled.

Love Actually is one of those movies that has several different storylines running at once — all these narrative threads that make up the main story and the characters kind of know each other in one way or another. I mean it can be fairly complicated for even a sane person to follow. Imagine showing that movie to a bunch of crazies. It was mental. Literally. The scene where the characters are pretending to have sex, working as stunt doubles on a movie set... Wowsers. It was a major trigger for me.

I started to panic. I didn't know what was real. Was I having an episode and imagining this scene? Did the people on the screen actually have their clothes on or not? Was it all part of the film for real or was it all in my head? I had a mini-breakdown right there on my plastic chair and had to be escorted back to my dorm by the Occupational Therapist on duty. I still think it was a stupid choice of movie to screen in a mental ward. Like seriously people: Get your shit together.

Most of the time it was difficult to differentiate between the nurses and the patients. Not just in my mind either. In real life that was actually the case. Everyone kind of just blended into one inside those walls. I guess that was the nature of the beast.

I did have a favourite nurse though. I remember feeling relieved whenever she was rostered on because her presence managed to dissolve my anxiety and fear. She had flame red hair and a big wide smile, and she treated everyone the same. With care and dignity we were all equal in her eyes and there was no room whatsoever for judgement. She only dealt in patience and compassion and she radiated a kind of peacefulness. Unbeknown to her she offered me great hope, leaving a significant mark on who I would one day become.

When you're a Ward of the State, you have to eventually appear in court so the judge can listen to evidence and determine whether or not

you are a danger to yourself or to others.
Based on the findings presented at the hearing,
you can be released back into 'normal society'.
Let's just say that my first court hearing
didn't go down so well.

At this point I still had no idea of the bigger
picture. There were times when I genuinely felt
fairly sane, but other times when I'd become
very good at pretending. I'd do something
like pour all my meds down the bathroom sink
(forgetting there was nowhere to hide in that
place) and then they would proceed to push the
court date back again. I was trying to be on my
best behaviour, without understanding what
I was actually *behaving* for.

One day my mother came to visit. She wanted
to prep me and talk through the upcoming court
appearance. She asked me how I was doing that
day, and I told her I'd become obsessed with washing
my hands. Like, every five minutes kinda deal.

"I think you should stop doing that," she said.
"If you want to get out of here, it probably
won't work in your favour."

In the end, it took more than obsessive
hand-washing to bring me down. On the morning
of the court hearing I had my first full-blown
psychotic breakdown in weeks. It was brutal.

A doctor came to assess me, to determine whether I was fit to appear in court. He was Indian, but this time he wasn't God or any of his disciples. He was the devil. Coming to kidnap me. I was a young Indian girl, and he was coming to attack me. So that ended the court case right then and there.

My memories from the time in hospital aren't as clear as those leading up to arriving there. I would certainly attribute that to the amount of medication I was taking, as well as the fact that I was surrounded by other mentally ill people every minute of every day. I'm sure I have blocked a lot of the memories out, to be honest; it's not somewhere I ever long to revisit. When you are absorbing that much energy from those around you it becomes almost impossible to determine what is yours and what is theirs, whose trauma belongs to who, and how much of it you're imagining and how much of it is real. If you ask me, one definition of insanity is putting someone insane into an *insane* environment... it makes no sense, right?

What chance did any of us have to start learning to live a more normal existence when we are all wandering around a maze of concrete corridors, each of us experiencing our own intense levels of psychosis and trauma? We literally fed off each other's insanity.

It was crazy town alright. And I wasn't leaving any time soon.

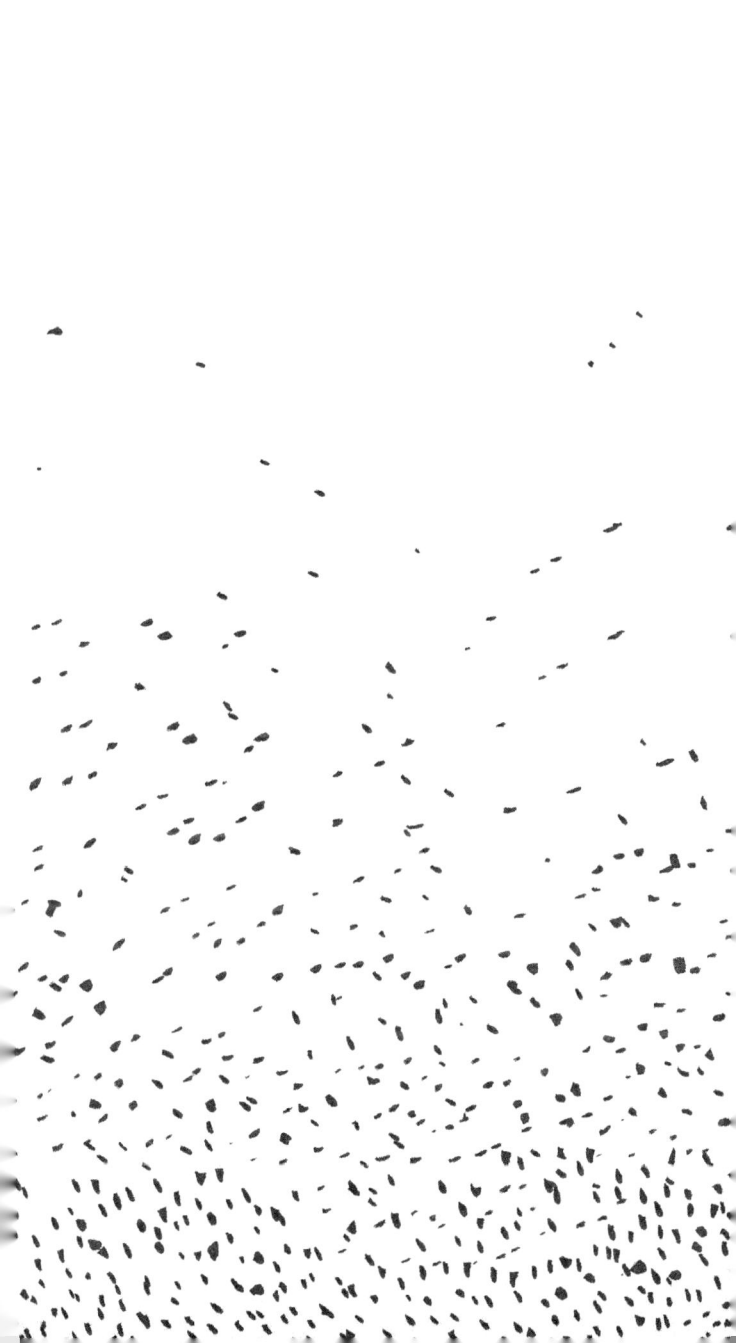

SMALL CAPPUCCINO

CHAPTER SEVEN

The lowest point in my newfound sanity was getting genuinely excited about being able to order my own coffee at the corner store. It was also the highest point in my recovery because I finally had the capability to actually speak for myself. It was the most I had to offer the world at that time, and to this day it has given me incredible perspective.

Eventually I left the public psychiatric hospital and transferred to the mental ward at the local private facility. It did take me a long time to feel comfortable enough to consider a change in my surroundings. I was frightened of the outside world and where the new me would fit into it. The court hearing passed and I was freed from the custody of the state. Mum reassured me it would be much nicer and more safe in my new ward, so I gave the private hospital a chance. *Like living in a bloody mental ward could be nice.*

From my new room I sat staring out the window that looked over the hospital car park, the hours ever so slowly passing by. I watched people being wheeled in chairs, or led by the arm, and helped in and out of cars. Where had they come from and where were they going? I wondered.

**Everyone seemed fragile, like they'd float
away at a gust of wind.**

The window was locked,

tightly shut,

unbreakable glass.

I couldn't smash my way through

or breathe the fresh air.

We went on 'excursions' every few days, shuffling
down the street to the local supermarket to buy a
chocolate bar, chaperoned by the occupational
therapist on duty. We were a sad old bunch:
a group of psych patients wandering aimlessly
along the foot path with glassy eyes peering
down at the pavement. Each of us in our own
dark reality, attempting to keep one foot
in front of the other. I was encouraged by
my doctors to attend the group art therapy
sessions that were held across the garden from
my room. Apparently they were 'good for my
concentration levels and sociability'.

It was debilitating to think that the highlight of my life had become cutting and pasting like a child. I remember carefully sticking patterned paper and coloured shapes onto a small wooden box that would become my 'treasure chest'. My family celebrated my works of art as some kind of sanctimonious achievement. I was so sarcastic and cynical about my situation, but when the sarcasm wore off all that was left was immense pain. Overweight and deeply depressed, sitting inside the walls of a psychiatric hospital making papier mâché and expected to be proud of how far I had come. It was degrading. I was begrudgingly attending these activities that were supposedly good for me, but really all I wanted was to go to sleep and never wake up.

That was my life.

My girlfriend would come to visit me fairly regularly in the private hospital, the one who had witnessed my dramatic goodbye all those months ago. She'd paint my nails whilst telling me all about what was going on in the real world, even though I was never fully present to listen. In fact, most of the time I remained unable to recognise who she even was. One random day she sat cross-legged on the end of my bed, flipping through a glossy magazine while I slept.

I opened my eyes, blinking, and turning my head from side to side on the pillow. As I began to awaken the first thing I noticed was the room appeared to be different. It was bright and light, not the sterile shades of white and grey I'd become so accustomed to. I could hear the gentle rustle of turning pages.

"It's so good to see you!" I said to her as I propped myself up from the pillows, pushing the blankets slowly from my legs and curling my knees up toward my chest. My movements were still slow and uncoordinated but my mind felt sharper than it had been for a long time.

My friend smiled at me. "Hey you." She might have been there for hours or perhaps she had sat there every day; I wouldn't have known it. Because the real *Emma* hadn't seen her in months.

I felt like I had broken the surface.

Something had definitely shifted inside my brain, as if I was coming out of the fog. It was a genuine, physical feeling. *I felt different.* The memories started fading immediately, melting away into the recesses of my subconscious mind like a poisonous gas. Colours were brighter, sounds were sharper, faces whole and tinged with the pink of fresh blood pumping through veins. I'd finally come up for air.

Surprisingly, the vivid memories of my psychotic episodes have remained far stronger than the memories I have from my time at the private psychiatric unit. And strangely, from that exact point of resurfacing, as in the day my girlfriend was at the end of my bed, my memories of life in general leading up to my breakdown became patchy. I am certain there is a scientific explanation for the big missing gaps, a side effect no doubt from all of the medication. The doctors had nurtured my brain with all kinds of medication in order to regain a certain level of stability, which in turn seemed to wipe everything else away. Once the fog started to lift the medication was designed to keep my brain functioning at a slow yet stable level, closely controlled and manipulated regularly by a team of trusted psychiatrists.

I was forced to come to terms with what my life looked like now and as I faced that reality I was blanketed by immense sadness. I was engulfed in a thick black cloud as I sank lower and lower into a deep depression. I felt like a stranger in my own skin; I even looked different, almost unrecognisable. My body was frumpy and my eyes lacked any spark. Underneath all the extra weight, I felt empty. Completely drained. I'd say it was the hardest time of all — the last few weeks in that private hospital, nurses coming and going 24 hours a day, feeling desperately sorry for myself, pulling the covers up over my head to hide who I had become from the outside world. I slept most of the time, this time by conscious choice, as I was finally fully aware of exactly *where* I was. And I hated it.

When people visited me, thankfully their faces weren't zombies anymore, but they looked at me with a pitying gaze that was inescapable.

"Look at you," their eyes seemed to say. "Who would've thought you of all people would end up like this."

I shrivelled deeper under my crisp hospital bed sheets deeply ashamed. And to make matters worse, some of the occupational therapists and psychologists on my ward had accompanying students. Students that I had personally been to school and university with, and now I was their actual patient! The shame was unbearable. *Kill. Me. Now.*

After six more weeks of hospital care I moved back home and became an outpatient. My newfound sanity that my family had so desperately prayed for arrived, but the truth was it was a different kind of debilitating in itself. I wasn't able to work, I had lost almost all of my friends, I didn't have a valid driver's license, and I was granted a disability pension. I was a puffy, dependent, incapable mass of uselessness. It's a heartbreaking time to remember. I turned 21 and the last thing I wanted to do was celebrate.

Everything I had, I didn't have anymore. Everything I'd once looked forward to, I didn't have to look forward to anymore. My family took me out for dinner and I sat there, a broken and swollen mess at the end of the table wishing I would never see another birthday. I wanted nothing more than to be forgotten.

My parents weren't a whole lot happier than me. My mother was experiencing her own level of depression in the form of intense exhaustion and stress. Months of her life had essentially been on hold while she cared for me, and then visited me daily in the hospital, and now she had me at home again, as a heavily depressed outpatient on antipsychotic meds. Her relationship with my father was over and she was all but alone in the family home she had worked tirelessly to create. This was definitely one of the most challenging times in mum's life.

One morning as an outpatient, mum pulled up outside the local cafe and I walked in and ordered a coffee, all by myself. I hadn't communicated with anyone other than doctors, nurses, psychologists, and my fellow psych patients for a very long time. And I hadn't experienced a customer service exchange with a normal human member of the public since before I became ill, so to be able to say

"Hi, can I have a small cappuccino?"

was a significant thing. I was so proud of myself.
There was a moment when I observed myself
waiting for my coffee at the other end of the
counter, and I distinctly remember thinking,
"Look at you, Em. Ordering your own coffee.
Go you!" It was a tiny triumph but at the time
it meant so much. Looking back now it is by
far one of my most humbling of memories.
It brings me to tears to think that *that* was
the state of my existence.

I slept a lot, I ate a lot, and I stayed inside a lot.
Days turned into weeks, with nowhere to go
and nothing to do. It was a random Wednesday
morning and I was alone in my bedroom when
I heard it. The familiar music blaring from the
next-door neighbour's stereo. I was instantly
unravelled by the pain of nostalgia. Flooded by
the memories of *him*, my body took over as
I shook with tears of grief. I missed him.
I missed his presence. His love. *Our love*.
Our toxic love that no one understood.
Playing in the background of my emotions was
this particular song. A song that brought me to
tears every time I heard it. Be it in the hospital,
in the car, in the grocery store, it didn't matter
where I was at the time, hearing the familiar
melody instantly transported me to a different

place. The place where he was, gently strumming that familiar tune on his acoustic guitar.

I remember one day hearing it over the crackling hospital speakers, just days after being admitted into the public psych ward. Even in the midst of deep psychosis, when I had zero concept of reality, I heard that song and the instant memory of him made me inconsolable. It was deep, tumultuous heartbreak and being stuck in my illness left me with no words to articulate it; only the feeling remained. My body had absorbed that song when we were together, and somewhere buried deep within my subconscious, I associated that exact melody with him and a moment of real beauty amid the chaos that was our tortured relationship.

He had been gone for just over one year and was recently back in town when fate stepped in. My girlfriend literally ran into him one random afternoon at the beach. They each stopped in their tracks as recognition dawned. The first thing he asked her was, "How's Em?" She was taken aback in realising that he knew absolutely nothing of what had become of me.

It didn't take him long to find the courage to come and visit. He knocked at the front door. My mother answered. I almost died when I clocked eyes on him. I guess part of me thought I'd never *ever* be seeing him again. Yet here he was.

He walked into our living room and stood in front of me. I was a mental patient who had almost doubled in size since he'd last seen me; I didn't even look the same. *I wasn't the same*. But he saw straight through all that. Almost instantly he became my connection back to a time when I felt somewhat lovable.

He represented familiarity, and familiar was safe.

We got back together. We became virtually inseparable. He worked away a lot and when he was in town he either was at home with me at my place or I was with him at his. I was the common ground between mum and him, although they had never really gotten along in the past, they did now because they were both equally as invested in me and my health. My mother could see that his life was back on track, and she knew that he saw through the surface of my illness — the puffy, heavily depressed shadow of my former self — to the real me. Mum understood that through everything it was hard for me to assimilate back into normal life. And at the time I honestly didn't want to do life at all. But since he came back around, I did kind of want to do life with him. There was hope. He gave me hope.

Within weeks, I got pregnant. It was a huge shock and it made no sense. I was still ingesting a daily cocktail of anti-psychotic medication and my body was not functioning normally. I was dazed and confused. And pregnant.

I arrived home from a walk one sunny afternoon and was confronted by a full-on intervention staged by my family, with the mental health crisis team backing them up for support. Everyone was deeply concerned for my future. They were genuinely worried about the need to come off my high-dose medication if I were to persist with the pregnancy. It was likely that without meds I could lose my mind again, so there was little more conversation to be had: I was deemed unfit to be a mother. The pregnancy was terminated.

We stayed away from each other for a while. He thought it would be best that way. Although from time to time we saw each other, locked in a twisted and toxic embrace that neither of us could escape, nor did we really want to.

Then I got pregnant again.

Of course it remained to make no sense. This time I was even on the pill and I was still dosed up on medication. Yet there it was, a bold positive result on the stick in my shaking hand indicating another tiny fertilised egg had broken through.

I refused to sign the forms.
Everyone was beyond ropeable:

"You can't do it, Em. You have to sort this out; you are being completely irresponsible not considering the future for your unborn child, and besides that, it's just not a good thing for you. What about your mental health? Your circumstances are no different to what they were six weeks ago!"

My mother was furious. Furious and frightened that she would soon be responsible for a psychotic patient *and* her offspring.

"If this is what you want, you are going to have to leave."
She was at her wits end and saw a future of chaos, as a single working mother in her 50's, caring for not only me, but for my baby too. I completely understood that. But no way in hell was I backing down. I had prayed and prayed and *prayed* for a saviour, for a miracle. With each day that passed I refused with whatever strength I could muster to accept the prognosis of a future shattered by episodes of insanity. My faith was the one thing that couldn't be taken away. And as crazy as it may sound still to the very day, I *knew* in my heart this baby was the answer to my prayers.

"It may not make any sense to you or to anyone, but this is what I want." I replied, defiant.

"You aren't fit to know what you want."
My mother was frustrated and full of fear.

"This time you can't convince me mum. This is my life and this is my decision. And no one is taking it away from me."

I wasn't going to back down; already I could feel a new sense of determination and strength kicking in.

"Fine, then you can go! Go to him!"
She stormed out of the living room.

I took off out the back door. It was a cool Autumn day and the wind pierced through my pale blue jumper. I reached for the hood and pulled it firmly down over my eyes. I gritted my teeth and swallowed the massive lump in my throat. Why couldn't anyone understand? I knew I had to have this baby. I also knew it didn't make any sense. I was frustrated and confused. I didn't know where to go. I didn't know what to do.

I knocked on his door. Reluctantly he let me in. I think he too truly feared raising a baby alone if I once again fell victim to the claws of psychosis, but thankfully he let me stay. Within a few days my dad showed up. Again with tears streaming down his face, he carefully unloaded my belongings from the back of his ute. My father was under strict instructions to leave my things and the situation exactly where it was. I'll never forget that day.

For the first time in my life I felt there was no one left to lean on.

For a while it was a living hell. My mental state remained to be maintained by an array of medication, and the doctors strongly advised that I shouldn't be put under any stress. It wouldn't be good for my brain. I was way too fragile to withstand any unnecessary pressure. In light of all that, against the doctor's recommendations, I decided I wanted to wean myself off the meds. So under what was perceived as somewhat reluctant medical supervision, I came off the drugs. Six months pregnant, living smack bang in the middle of one hell of a volatile relationship, the stress piled up yet I remained focused and committed to my one and only goal. To keep my sanity.

It's hard to explain but I *knew*, I just knew in my heart that I could become a mother and that I wouldn't ever fall ill again. I was about seven months pregnant when once again something shifted inside my mind. I again experienced a significant resurfacing moment, I felt like I'd broken through once more. I remember talking to my sister Peta on the phone that day and she said,

"Wow, you sound different. You sound like the old you.
I think I might even have my sister back."

She couldn't contain her excitement.

Our relationship had never been the same since my illness. I remember the feeling that random day. It came on strong. I felt so clear, *mentally clear.* And by god was I going to do everything in my power to make sure the clarity remained.

I knew I had been given a second chance and I remember thinking, "Whatever you do Em, *do not* stuff this one up." It wasn't just about me anymore. I had stood alone in my decision to bring an innocent life into the world, and now I had to step up and take full responsibility for my life, and for his life, for *both* of us. There was a lot riding on it, but I honestly didn't feel any pressure. Only hope for the future.

I felt a surge of motivation, as if I'd been struck by a lightning bolt. I finally had the energy in the tank and taking care of my health, both mentally and physically, was no longer negotiable. It was mandatory.

I exercised most days taking long walks on the beach in the sunshine, filling my lungs with the fresh salty air as the waves rolled in. I even worked up the courage to join an evening

Pilates class. I gave up eating junk food and became conscious of all that I fed my body and my mind. I realised there was such a thing as 'mood food', that what I put into my physical self directly affected my mental state too. I spent countless days and nights alone in my thoughts. But this time they were hopeful thoughts; I finally had something to look forward to. Above all else I valued my sanity, and peace was my highest priority during this time. What delivered me to peace faster than anything else was sunlight, moving my body mindfully (I became a Pilates convert), practicing deep breathing as often as I could, and surrounding myself with the people who loved me the most. I kept a gratitude journal and I counted my blessings every single day. My 'pregnancy milestone diary' was my most prized possession as I carefully recorded the finest of details to ensure this baby knew what his existence meant to me.

Since coming off my medication I didn't have so much as a hint of psychosis. My recovery from the chronic episodes was virtually deemed miraculous, but never for a second did I believe that. I am no miracle, but I did often pray for one as you know.

In November of that same year, the year I was 21 — and really still a baby myself — I brought another baby into this world. My son, Gabriel.

GABRIEL

CHAPTER EIGHT

I arrived at the birthing suite just after midnight. It was a packed house that night, (and according to one of the midwives on duty who greeted me as I doubled over whaling in pain mid-contraction in the entry hall), "as the last one to arrive here honey, don't expect to be the first to deliver. We are run off our feet tonight, there's almost no room at the inn." And off she literally ran. And arrive my baby did. First. To everyone's surprise the labour lasted less than forty minutes. It was fast and extremely painful, but most importantly completely uncomplicated. And it's funny that right from the get go, that's exactly how my beautiful firstborn son has been. Uncomplicated.

Giving birth changed me.

And I know all mothers would say that. I had walked through a doorway and there was no turning back. The responsibility dawned on me, I was now needed 24/7 by a living, breathing little human. Motherhood might have arrived early, but it arrived at exactly the right time. In all honesty, my dream for the three of us to become a happy family faded quickly. I knew the relationship long term could not survive, but the physical logistics were more difficult to figure out. It took some time to break away. We were naturally still involved in each other's lives, because after all, we shared a child now. But in our hearts we both knew the end was near, and soon it was over. I became a single mother. And I was honestly relieved.

I still manage to hold onto what I learned during that tumultuous time. I learned the importance of taking the high road, and how not to sweat the small stuff. I learned how to mentally detach myself from situations of stress by taking long deep breaths. I learned the value of being non-reactive and the value of speaking less and listening more. But most of all I learned *a lot* about faith. Faith taught me that in relationships, it is critical to not only believe in each other but to first and foremost believe in yourself, holding a space for both of you to grow from. Back then I certainly believed I could be better. And better one day I would be.

Gabe and I moved back in with my mother for a time but it wasn't long before she took a job in the city which meant she had to leave town. My family support was very limited because both my dad and sisters had already moved away. Gabriel's grandparents (on his dad's side) were a beacon of light during that time, and they still remain to be to this very day. Always unwavering in their commitment to their grandson, and forever respectful of me and my decisions. There is a glorious simplicity about the two of them, a real sense of home. As much as Gabe has filled their lives with joy and purpose, the stability and unconditional love they have offered me over the years has greatly contributed to who I have become.

Gabriel was like the catalyst that repaired so much brokenness. His effortless ability to heal was apparent right from the start. I knew back then, all I needed to do was to nurture and protect his light, and then from that same place I could make my decisions wisely. I took his lead and faced the difficult calls head on. His spirit affected mine, and I consciously chose love over fear. I was constantly reminded that so many people loved Gabriel enormously. And that loving part in all of them deserved to feel love reciprocated, and peace as well. Gabe taught me what it truly means to be fearless. He taught me to forgive. He showed me the way back to living from the heart.

I remember resting in hospital in the hours

just after he was born. A stark white room so different to those I'd become accustomed to in the previous year. Helium balloons floated near the ceiling. "It's a boy!" in cursive bright blue lettering. Fresh flowers on the tableside next to my bed. I had my knees bent up under the blankets and I held his two tiny hands as his itty-bitty body reclined on my thighs. During a moment of stillness, of silence, with no visitors or midwives bustling in and out, we stared at each other. Breathing together in sync we locked eyes. And for a prolonged and mystical moment, his eyes became those of an old man's, deep and wise, telling a lifetime's worth of stories as he gazed right back at me. It wasn't my frightening imagination this time, it was real. He was an old soul and as his face changed for that moment in time, I felt reassurance, I felt a new kind of safe.

During the times when I was emotionally overcome or strung out, as any ultra-busy single mother would get like from time to time, I would creep into his bedroom at night and climb into his little toddler bed. Just to be near his soft sleeping energy for a moment would bring me comfort. I naturally gravitated towards him because even in his sleep he could take me by the hand and show me what I'd forgotten, what I needed to *remember*. By focusing on Gabriel it was much easier to let go. The veil of darkness and fear would lift once more and out of my anxiety came peace.

Gabe took his first steps in Scotland. The only way to make a clean break was to leave the country. Things were really difficult with his father, heart-wrenchingly so. We didn't have a normal life. It was like living in a fish bowl. As a single mum I worked three jobs to support us, and somehow also studied at university. I was exhausted and overworked, very thin again and not really looking after myself. My life was dominated by children's books and movies, Thomas the Tank Engine, The Wiggles, Bananas in Pyjamas. My entire life was consumed with work and motherhood, and in many ways I couldn't have been happier. I had my own space and at some level I was free.

Although this kind of life as a single mum brought its own array of challenges, my experience of severe mental illness had given me such a platform of perspective. I could constantly compare the state of my life in that moment to what it was like being in a hospital for the clinically insane. At least I could sleep in the safety of my own home without the risk of being potentially violated by Slim Shady in the middle of the night. At least no one was serving me boobs for dinner. At least the screaming inside my mind had stopped.

I would come home from work, play with my baby, bathe him, feed him and put him to bed. Then I'd finally get to enjoy a glass of wine and a moment of quiet reflection. Sitting on my back balcony I realised my former self would never have been able to even comprehend a life of such simplicity.

Although I was grateful to be out of the relationship with Gabe's father, by many standards I still wasn't whole-heartedly *living*. I was on auto-pilot a lot, just simply surviving the daily grind. I still felt greatly unsettled, unsure whether to move us to the city, to finish my degree, or to put down roots somewhere else. I definitely felt we needed a change in scenery. Maybe a holiday was what I needed. I hadn't really thought a great deal about traveling the world and I originally thought that having a baby virtually made it well out of the question. But then one day out of nowhere I realised I had managed to put away enough money to go overseas. There was nothing stopping us. So when Gabriel was 14 months old we set off on a European adventure. And it changed my life.

A 21-year-old, rake-thin girl with a baby and a backpack.

My sister Han joined us. We had an absolute ball the three of us together. I can't begin to describe the feeling of freedom that surrounded me the minute I got off the plane at Heathrow Airport. There was this sense of ultimate renewal in the air. Finally with the distance from home, I could fully exhale. I could be myself.

Gabe's big brown eyes lit up at the sight of the famous bright red buses weaving in and out of traffic along bustling Oxford Street. It was in the middle of Hyde Park on an icy cold February afternoon that he got to touch snow for the first time. Dressed in a navy-blue coat with his hood tightly fastened around his little chin, he squealed in sheer delight as his chubby fingers froze, busily shaping mismatched snowballs.

Whilst exploring Edinburgh Castle Gabe took his first steps, regularly toppling over on the uneven cobblestones underfoot. He was never down for long, clinging to my jeans to steady himself and regain balance before toddling off once more. He wasn't afraid to fall over.

He slept soundly in my backpack as I stood in awe at the top of the Eiffel Tower as the view below took my breath away. The sprawling city of love stretched out before me as far as the eye could see and time stood still for a silent blissful moment as I was overcome with gratitude that literally filled me up from my toes to the top of my head. It was right then and there in Paris that I realised how far I'd really come, in more ways than one.

The eclectic sites, smells and sounds home to Las Ramblas Barcelona didn't startle Gabe at all, not even for a second. He was fascinated by the loud street performers, artists and bird aviaries that lined the famous colourful stretch.

It was a feast for the senses bordering on sensory overload at times, and so for the break I needed I decided we'd make the massive hike by foot to the top of the vibrant Spanish city. It was there nestled amongst the bright blue mosaic statues, home to Gaudi's Park Guell, where we relished in the calm. Gabe played for hours, until sunset in fact. It was heaven, and a feeling I will never ever forget.

Gabriel always had such an unwavering patience. It was that patience that made our traveling experience actually possible. He really did make it uncomplicated, in fact it was easy. He was happy day after day to kick back and take it all in from his seat perched high up on my back.

The Trevi Fountain, St Peter's Basilica, the Spanish Steps — we witnessed Rome in all it's glory. At the Colosseum we had a slight wardrobe malfunction in that Gabe peed through his nappy resulting in his pants being completely soaked. Of course that had to be the day that I'd forgotten to pack spare clothes for our day trip, so we were forced to join the group tour with him wrapped in a blanket. I still joke with Gabe now that he was a pant-less Gladiator. Not everyone can claim they visited The Colosseum without their pants.

In a Venice restaurant he slept soundly under the table. Curled up so warm and cosy in a makeshift bed on the floor as Han and I ate spaghetti, drank red wine and shared a whole lot of laughs well into the night. It was like a dream. There I was, barely a woman, without a care in the world, experiencing the trip of a lifetime, and never once did my son hold me back. Gone were my nightmares, this was heaven on earth.

We were away for two months and when we returned home all I wanted was that feeling back. I did everything in my power to be able to return. This time the plan was to move to London. I worked hard for a year, and just after Gabriel's second birthday our plan was to head off again. My cousins lived in the UK and there was the opportunity to put down roots, start a new life from the ground up. A change even better than a holiday.

Well that was the plan anyway. But I had forgotten for a second that life doesn't always go to plan. As fate would have it, six teeny weeks before we were due to fly out, I met Jase.

It was Anzac Day and Gabe was visiting his grandparents for the public holiday. I had made plans to go out with a girlfriend. I remember feeling really tired that afternoon and I knew the scene out on the town would be packed and messy. I really didn't want to go out but I had promised the girls I'd show up and I don't like letting people down.

We walked into the pub and I saw him immediately. He was dressed in a fitted bright green shirt, with a killer smile and friendly blue eyes, but above all else the first thing I actually noticed were his arms. *Oh, dear lord the man worked out.* Now I'm not going to lie and say it was love at first sight; I was definitely intrigued by him, but I was also very judgemental. Honestly, I thought he was one of *those guys.* Those gorgeously charming, smooth talking, bench-press-loving, super fit guys, with a supersized ego to match. Not usually am I one to stereotype, but in this case I was completely guilty.

He was sitting at the bar talking to the manager, who happened to be a good friend of mine. His eyes met mine as I approached the bar and ordered drinks.

"Em, have you met my brother Jason?"

I reached out and shook his hand. Looking awkwardly at my bar manager friend I remember thinking to myself, "how did I not know you had a brother?"

"What are you drinking?" I casually asked Jase.

He held up a water bottle.
"Oh, no thanks. I don't drink."

"Right, so you're one of those guys... my body is a temple... I get it. Okay."
I rolled my eyes, turned to my friend and giggled. She smirked back at me.

"So, you're judging me because you think I am either appearance obsessed, or prefer drugs to beer, or both," Jason quipped back, meeting me smirk for smirk. *"Well for the record, I don't do drugs. But I do care about my body so I'm not a big drinker."*

The bass from the dance floor in the next room thudded under the bottom of my feet and up my shins to the crown of my head. My palms itched. I was being an arsehole because I was totally intimidated. His presence was intimidating and I kept expecting him to stop talking to me the minute a hot chick walked through the door.

"Cool, well I'm going outside for a cigarette."
I indicated to my friend, and grabbed
my purse from the bar top.

"Oh, you're a smoker. Also for the record, I'm not into it"
Jase was now the one full of judgement.

*"Wow mister judg-eeee. Well, if you must know, I wouldn't
call myself a full time smoker. I do enjoy the occasional
social one though when I'm drinking."*

Why all of a sudden did I feel compelled to tell him
everything? I automatically cared what he thought
of me. Damn it. I was annoying myself now.

He nodded and raised his eyebrows, still with
an infuriating smirk on his face like he knew
he was hot stuff and that I was flustered.

Outside I bumped into a friend. She started
going on and on about this guy she just saw
inside who was a total babe but she was way
too shy to talk to him. I offered to be her
wingman, I didn't have a problem playing cupid.
I followed her back into the bar and she pointed
out *the* guy, wearing a bright green shirt sitting
with a group of people in the far corner of the
bar. He was half-obscured by the people
playing pool at the table in the centre of the
room, but I knew exactly who she meant.

She was interested in Jason. My gut reaction said, "no way in hell am I setting her up with him." I was definite about that and it felt weird to be so certain. I mean up until that point I had absolutely zero interest in men. In many ways I was terrified of them. And besides that, I didn't even want to go out that night anyway.
Yet there I was really caring. I found myself frozen in the face of agreeing to set my friend up with this guy whom I had just met, whom I had absolutely no claim over, whom I was certain would have zero interest in me.

Meanwhile and annoyingly so, Jase knew exactly what was going on and he playfully backed me into a corner where I was forced to admit point blank to his face that I was interested in him. Talk about no holds barred. As humiliating as it could have been I just went for it. I think it was the most forward I have ever been in my life.

Jase and I ended up talking the night away, but in the pit of my stomach was Gabriel. With every hour of conversation that passed, I still hadn't mentioned him. I felt sicker by the second, and guilty. More and more guilty. Here I was, having a real, raw, beautiful conversation with someone who I almost instantly connected with, and I hadn't yet told him about my main man. I began questioning why I felt the need to keep my son a secret?

My self-esteem was at an all-time low. As a single mum I had taken myself 'off the shelf.' I was greatly afraid of meeting men because I felt like I came with a whole lot of extra responsibility. This wasn't a classic fairy tale, and I certainly wasn't a picture of perfect purity.

I wanted to be confident and outspoken about my beautiful little boy and I really wanted to be upfront with Jase, but to be frank, I never expected that we would talk any longer than ten minutes in a crowded noisy bar. I thought I'd never see this guy again, so the less he knew the better.

As Jase was driving me home hours later, the first light of dawn creeping over the horizon at the beach, I finally turned to face him from my place in the passenger seat. My palms were sweaty.

"I have to tell you something."
I was a bucket of nerves.

He smiled, that small smile bordering on a smirk, eyes glaring into my soul. *"What?"*

"I have a confession to make and I can't get out of the car until I tell you... I feel terribly guilty that I haven't told you yet. It should've been the first thing that I said."

He raised his eyebrows as if to say, *Go on.*

"I need you to know I'm a single mother, I have a son."

There was a moment of silence. I was too terrified to look at him, wringing my hands down in my lap over the seatbelt strap.

"I'm really glad you finally got that off your chest," he said cheekily. I looked up at his face. He was smiling. *"Do you think I don't already know that?"*

He started laughing and I soon joined him in the laughter. I felt like a first-class idiot. Of course Jason knew about Gabe. He had spent quite some time hearing about me from his brother — the manager of the bar, the good friend of mine — and unbeknown to me he'd already learned *a lot* about my story. Jason had played it cool but he'd known all along, watching me flounder and fall deeper into guilt with that smirk on his face, his idea of funny.

From that moment we began a passionate whirlwind love affair just six weeks before Gabe and I were due to leave the country for good. Talk about timing.

I kept thinking it was too good to be true, and naturally I was still nervous about having anyone new in my life. I was fairly resistant to begin with. After all, my life had been fairly complicated for a couple of long years. But Jason wasn't complicated, he was simple. He seemed solid. And I know that's what attracted me to him. There's something refreshing about meeting a grounded individual when you were once a total nut. I felt secure.

But I traded security for 'it's complicated.' We both still had a heap of growing to do. So in the May of that year, I packed my bags and we left for the airport. Pete was holding Gabe in her arms whispering her sweet goodbyes, and I stood directly opposite Jase and took a deep breath.

"I just want you to know that I love you, and I can't leave without saying those three little words. But I have to do this. I have to go. But that doesn't mean I don't love you." The gloves were off, I'd been brave enough to let my guard down and say it first. I didn't break his eye contact and I didn't hold back.

From the first second I clocked eyes on him Jason forced me to break barriers within myself. And in that moment standing right by the departure gates, he unravelled right in front of me. Tears streaming down his face, his whole body began to tremble. He came straight out with it, confessing his undying love for me and for Gabriel. I got quite a shock as I didn't expect it from someone who appeared to be so cool calm and collected. There was something incredibly comforting about his open and honest vulnerability in that moment. The man had the courage to show all of himself, to be his whole-self, and I greatly respected that. But I still had to let him go.

I turned away from him as I took Gabe's little hand and we walked through the security gates side by side. I'll never forget Pete calling me whilst we waited at the boarding gate, hissing that I'd left her out there to deal with Jase who was a fairly uncontrollable emotional wreck while she was not much more than a pile of rubbish herself. I think both Pete and I were flabbergasted by Jason's depth of love for me, I mean it had only been a matter of weeks since we'd actually met. But I had committed to myself for now, and for now it would remain just the two of us. My angel boy and me.

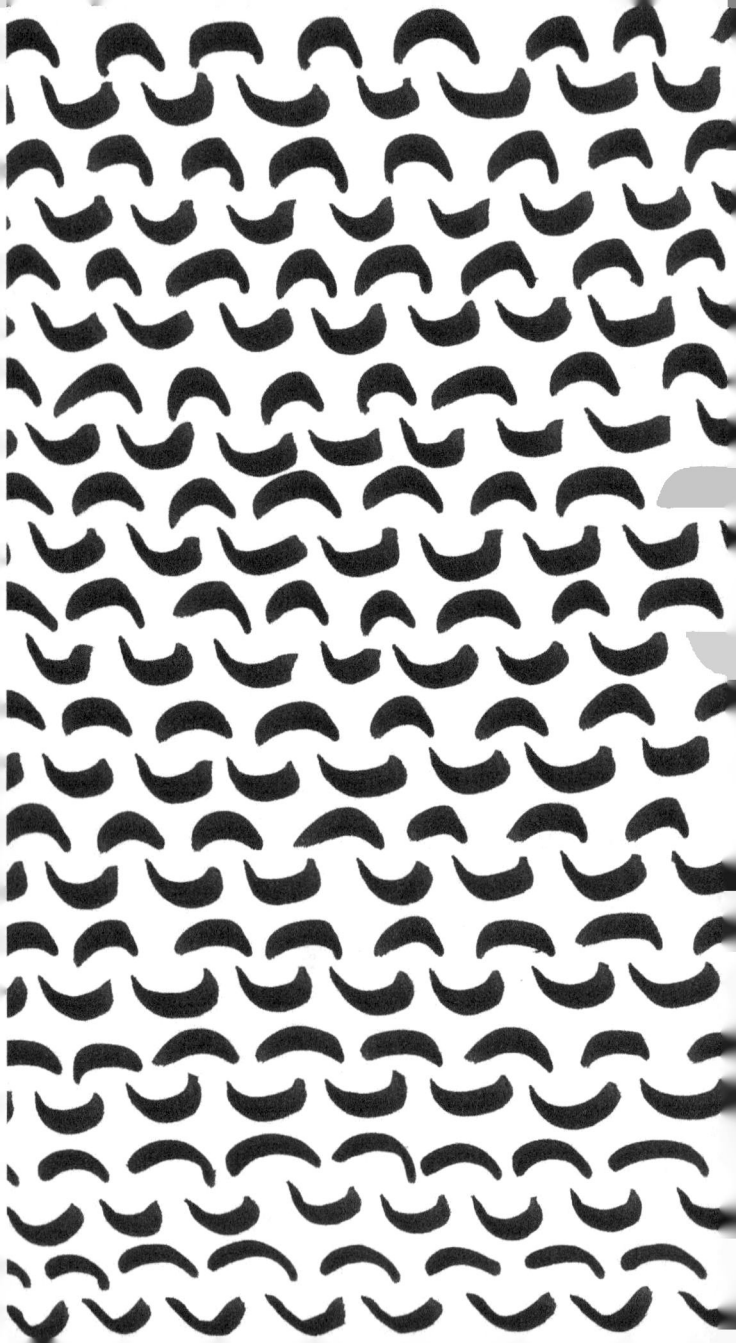

AN UNUSUALLY
LOUD HEARTBEAT

CHAPTER NINE

We left Australia and returned several months later. We didn't end up staying long term in London as planned. And within six months of being on the same soil, Jase and I were engaged. It was a whirlwind. And when I say whirlwind, I mean fucking whirlwind. We were married in October, just seven months after our engagement, and in the following August we welcomed our second son Riley into the world. Our new life together polarized that of before, in less than two years I went from being a single mother with a toddler, to a wife and mother of two gorgeous boys. Like always, it was water off a duck's back for Gabe, he adapted effortlessly to his new family environment. Me on the other hand, not so much.

When we first came back to Australia I had many reservations and conversations with Jase about Gabriel, "you can be involved in Gabe's life as little or as much as you like. But trust me, I have a strong feeling that he's the sort of kid you will want to get to know." Jason didn't hesitate. As he started to get to know Gabe it was no surprise that he found him to be the most inspiring little person he had ever met. It was incredible to observe the relationship between the two of them blossom. Gabe brought endless joy into Jason's life, and as the connection deepened it was clear Jase couldn't see his life spent in any other way. His Friday nights were now spent colouring in and playing toy trains, a far cry from his carefree party fueled weekends as a single man. Gabe in so many ways became the reality check Jase didn't realise he needed, until my little man came along and parked himself right in the centre of his life. Given the opportunity to step in as Gabe's father figure was a blessing Jase deeply treasured and he never once took it for granted.

For a while Gabe referred to him by his first name, he was "Jase" and I didn't encourage him otherwise. Like always, I took Gabe's lead. It was whatever made him feel the most comfortable that made me comfortable. But I'll never forget the day Gabe, completely off his own accord, called him "Dad." He had not long turned three and the festive season was upon us. We were heading out to a Christmas party and picking up Jase on our way. I was parked outside his house, the car idling, me in the driver's seat, Gabe in his car seat behind me.

The Wiggles Christmas Carols were playing
on the car stereo in the background.

"Mum, what are we doing?"

I turned the volume down.
*"We're waiting here darling because Jase
is getting ready and we are picking him up.
He's coming to the party with us"*

*"Oh. Right. But you mean my dad is getting ready.
Dad is coming to the party with us"*
Gabriel clearly corrected me.

From that point on, Gabe decided he had two dads, and he didn't question it, not even for a second. He thought he was the luckiest little dude in the world. The finer details didn't matter to him back then, and funnily enough — they still don't. As long as everyone was happy, Gabe was happy. His effortless ability to roll with the punches remains to inspire me every day as it's so far from my natural state. I question on the regular how I could have possibly brought such a calm human being into this world?

I've never been one to adjust to change easily. It's only been through the writing of this book that I have realised an underlying common theme in my life. A common theme which has bubbled away below the surface for as long as I can remember. The common theme I'm referring to is: anxiety. Anxiety can trick you into feeling out of control and helpless. Helplessness generates nervousness and in turn creates more anxiety. It really is a vicious cycle. I'm damn sure the anxiety (or common theme) in my life is related to my ridiculously high expectations of myself formed in childhood. It's the whole *not-attempting-to-walk-until-I-can-run* scenario rearing its perfectionist head. I've always preferred to be certain of situations, to know what to expect so that then I can best prepare. In Mark Manson's best-selling book 'The Subtle Art of Not Giving a Fuck', he says that

"The more you try to be certain about something, the more uncertain and insecure you will feel (*cue anxiety).

But the converse is true as well: the more you embrace being uncertain and not knowing, the more comfortable you will feel in knowing what you don't know."

And there I was again berating and beating myself up for my lack of preparation for married life. I mean how do you prepare for something you know nothing about? My anxiety and chronic perfectionism landed me again on struggle street. Midway into our first year of marriage, having not long given birth to my second son, I found myself in a deep hole of depression. Aaaaaagain.

I remember sitting across from my doctor in her office attempting to explain how stupid I felt. Here I was with a somewhat 'dream life.' The life I had least expected to be living, with a husband who loved me, a beautiful son, and a healthy baby, and yet I was miserable.

"I should be so happy. I have absolutely nothing to complain about. Yet I feel terrible. I am so sad all the time and all I want to do is pull the covers up over my head and cry. I have no reason to be like this. I should be overjoyed. I should be happy. I should be loving my life. I should be feeling everything that I'm not."

"Firstly, you need to drop the word 'should' from your vocabulary Em", my doctor responded with care. "I don't believe you are expected to feel a certain way at all. This is a huge adjustment, completely new territory, and you have gone through *a great deal* over the past few years. Suddenly becoming a wife and fulfilling your part in a new marriage can be challenging for the best of us. Plus you've just had a baby for goodness sake. You must stop beating yourself up."

My doctor was concerned about my symptoms of depression, and considering my history of psychosis, she felt it was best to prescribe some meds for a while. That in itself was a low point, I hadn't taken any medication for at least five years. But I was grateful for her advice and I was determined to feel better.

Opening up to Jase about my past was daunting. He didn't know a lot about my history, and I certainly hadn't come to accept all of it quite yet. Shame was my silencer and part of me really didn't want to talk about it. But the other part of me wanted to be entirely honest and upfront, all the while I was shit scared of his judgement and potential rejection.

What if he saw me as a crazy person and wanted nothing to do with me?

What if he decided it was all too hard?

What if I was too much of a risk for his future?

All of these questions circulated inside my head.

When I did finally work up the courage to tell him the whole truth, his reaction couldn't have been further from my fears. He was compassionate and patient and didn't hold back in his love and admiration for who I had become. Unlike many people, psychosis wasn't unknown to Jase. A good friend of his had experienced a psychotic breakdown many years ago and he remembered firsthand how frightening it was. He said it was "confronting and eerie" witnessing a friend in such a far-out state of mind, and he was deeply saddened by the stigma and shame that accompanied his mate's suffering. Unfortunately Jason's friend wasn't ever able to recover, leaving Jase with a yearning to better understand mental illness.

The part that inspired him the most about my history was the fact I had made a conscious choice to not let my past take hold of my future. I worked hard to detach myself from it. I chose to leave my old life behind in many ways, and I was determined to keep my new life unaffected by the times of compulsive valium popping and psychiatric units.

It was true that a huge part of me consciously no longer identified with the former (ill) version of myself. But this didn't just happen overnight. It took *a lot* of self-work. Originally I wasn't expected to recover from my psychotic illness — the science and the stats pointed to a life on disability support welfare. However I point-blank refused to accept a life that looked that way. It just wasn't meant for me. A little spark within started my recovery process all those years ago and it never went out. As easy as it could've been to stay down, I made the hardest choice of all — to get the hell back up and fight.

The trauma of psychosis did leave me constantly monitoring my mental state though, so when the familiar cloud of depression began to linger on the edges of my life once more, I was more than a little concerned. It was as if in the moment of finally being able to relax, the trauma of my past resurfaced and started chipping away at me again.

There was only one road to take. I was going to have to *feel the feelings* and revisit the 'self-work.' For that, I needed help. I didn't hesitate to book in with a psychologist and the counselling sessions were invaluable. I was diagnosed with Post Traumatic Stress Disorder and treated with Cognitive Behaviour Therapy and meditation. The experience with my therapist at that time was invaluable and gave me a few more practical tools for my kit. Still to this day I regularly call upon those tools to maintain my mental wellbeing.

Forget the stereotype of honeymooner newlyweds... our early years of marriage were freaking tough. I was 26, Riley was one of those babies that screamed a lot, and there was only one word to describe our life: HECTIC. Jase and I had opened our first business together, a gym, and we were both heavily required to work in the business — it was long days and even longer nights with an unsettled baby who would only ever sleep for 45-minute intervals before the screaming kicked in again. I struggled to adjust to parenting this baby that I simply couldn't soothe. No matter how hard I tried Riley just wouldn't settle. He was (and remains to be) the polar opposite to Gabe. I would become more and more stressed and anxious and overtired, and so would my Riley. I was a ball of nervous energy, often dragging my feet, with dark circles around my eyes. I eventually became filled with deep resentment. For my baby, for my husband, for everyone and everything.

I leaned on Jason a lot at that time, the truth was I really needed him. Jase was committed, stepping in to bond with his infant son, relentlessly soothing his unhappy little soul night after night, even though it meant he too would become fragile with all the sleep deprivation and stress. It became evident after trying almost every single piece of advice, remedy and solution known to man — our newborn son would not sleep unless he could lay with his head near his father's heart. We discovered that Jase had an unusually loud heartbeat, so to make it possible for Riley to rest to its rhythm, we were forced to engage in a continuous cycle of 'breastfeed-and-pass-the-baby' as the night time hours slowly passed by. The struggle was real. I felt isolated. I missed my husband. And I was deeply affected by the lack of time I had for Gabe.

Ultimately my experience of life after Riley led me to launch my 'Mums Empowered' program. I set out to provide a safe place for new mothers to prioritise themselves and their health. In a society that preaches that women can 'have it all', but first they must 'be it all'...

housewife, mother, lover, career woman, all-round-shit-together-earth-moving-super-woman with a cracking body to match,

a mother actually being able to *practically* take care of her own needs can be virtually fucking impossible. When I was pregnant with Riley I fell into my own mother's trap of finding meaning and validity and self-worth in my work. I dove head first into managing the gym and working way too hard which meant stress and exhaustion — and it was no one's fault but my own. I personally had set the expectations and then I personally demanded that I meet them. That *was* me.

Soon after having Riley I realised I had a huge problem working within the fitness industry.

I felt ill-aligned in my work. It seemed too aesthetic, superficial and ego-driven, and I didn't feel mothers were greatly nurtured or represented in this space. I truthfully had never had much of an interest in the physical (the body) — the metaphysical, (or the mind and soul), was my calling. I felt a strange incongruence as a Personal Trainer, between my true values and the self at the time I was presenting to be. But also I knew that my clients respected and connected with me on a deeper level. I decided to change things up a little. I developed programs that were physiologically designed to improve strength and fitness levels, whilst maintaining the focus in the gym on brain health and the incredibly positive effects physical exercise has on one's mental state. I guess you could say I wasn't brave enough at the time to clearly articulate my values, but the women who formed the Mums Empowered community understood there was a lot more to me than their gym program. I deeply cared about how they felt about themselves, and it is something I proudly still stand for to this very day.

During Riley's infant years I did become depressed again and at times I found myself completely at the mercy of anxiety. I'd managed to disguise the internal struggle by being super 'busy.' But the truth was I was in pain and being a total bitch to myself. I constantly judged myself for not being able to press pause and

be present with my baby. The sleep deprivation only created more stress and no matter how hard I tried, I couldn't settle myself.
I struggled to give myself a break and often

I wanted to run away. Run far, far away.

Of course I couldn't run away. So drawing upon exactly what I needed at that hectic time in my life — a sense of community, mutual respect, support, honesty, endorphins, and me-time, my work soon became my therapy. And that's why Mums Empowered was able to thrive so successfully as a business. I encouraged women to understand the value of 'me time', making it possible for them to experience firsthand the endorphins, mental clarity and perspective physical exercise can deliver. I longed to accept myself for more than my body, and I wanted to inspire other women to do the same. We can be healthy and honour our earth suits, but to know that

what we truly have to offer goes far beyond our physicality,

that's where the real power lies. Through the simple act of giving to others I was able to receive what I needed the most — the ability to be compassionate and gentler with myself. Through true connection with others in the same boat as myself, my journey of healing continued.

During that time my mother became a rock for me again. We would sit and drink red wine on Friday nights and she would offer her words of encouragement. "Look at how far you've come Em." Her recollection of the trauma of years gone by never far from the forefront of her memory. We would laugh and cry about the past, and then converse for hours about spirituality (our most favourite topic), to then shake-it-off and call it a night. There's something beautiful about the way in which my family looks forward and gets on with things, we've always loved hard and we always move on.

Piece by piece, my ability to surrender, and my newfound wisdom (that I didn't have to prove myself to anyone) to be happy and peaceful and 'successful' ... I exhaled again and the stress melted away.

Just like his older brother, Riley in his own special way has taught me some huge lessons. He too gets anxious, is a total perfectionist, and is often outright hard on himself and others as a result. Riley offered me the opportunity to deconstruct his perfectionism, in turn renouncing my own, a process that has seen me face head-on the dangers of people pleasing. In a beautiful and often painstaking way, Riley's little existence called for a wholehearted conversation around my own struggle to be worthy. He has always been my pocket mirror, forcing me to become more self-aware, to grow, and to be more patient in life. I am so grateful that in Riley I have a little partner in crime on this quest for freedom, to hold me accountable, and to serve as my little reminder that: in our right minds we can achieve anything.

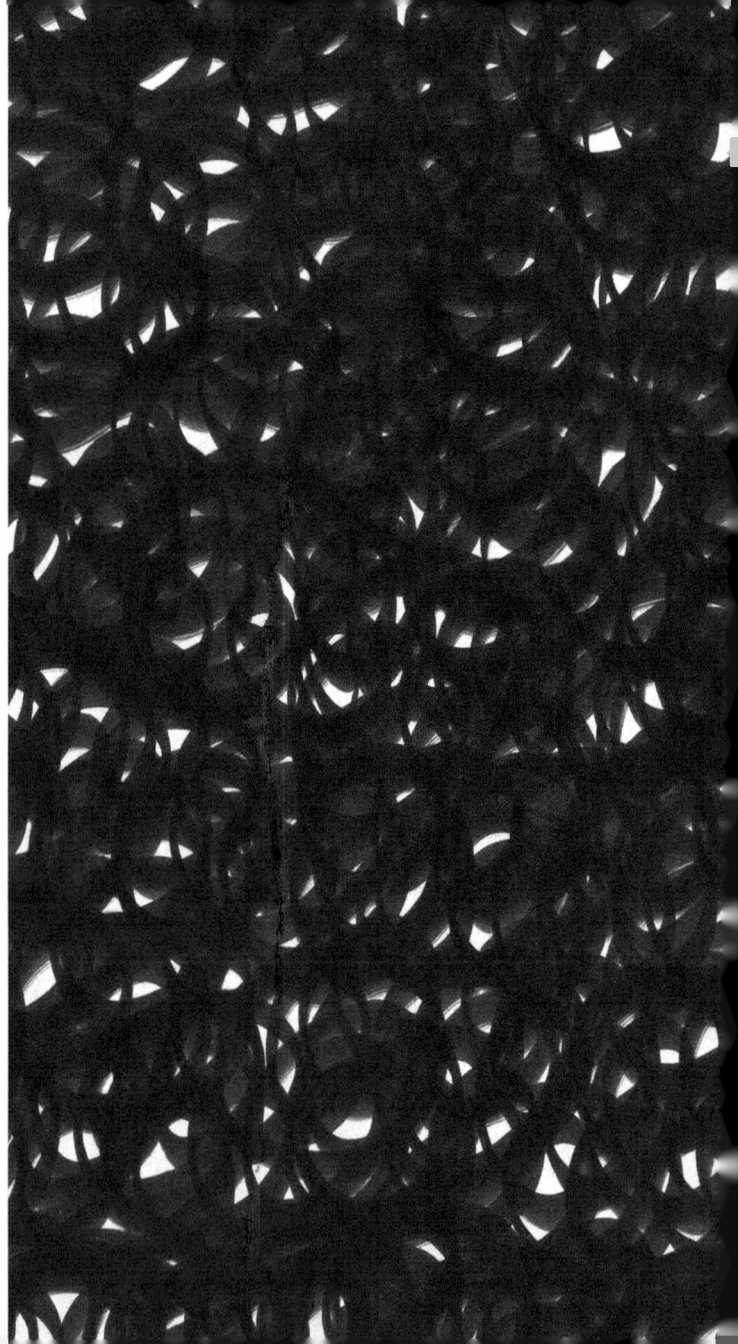

THE ELECTRICAL STORM

CHAPTER TEN

I turned 27 and things were traveling well.

My sister Peta had recently given me a little gem of wisdom: "before taking someone's advice, first look at the person giving it and decide whether they are someone you'd like to be like."

When I took on that little piece of wisdom, the world really did open up. I had been offered a great deal of advice over the years, and I think largely because of my need to please others, I was hasty to take on people's opinions as gospel. I finally got it. I started to do things differently. It didn't mean that I wasn't open to listen, but what it did mean was a new space to go within and trust myself, rather than continuously believing that someone other than myself knew the answers of my own heart.

I got my little girl. Lola Grace arrived. A beautiful baby girl born a few weeks early. Oh so tiny, yet healthy and perfect in every single way. And with her came the ultimate sense of renewal, a glorious opportunity to reset, to start again. When I looked at her I saw a version of my own little self, yet it was as if I was looking through a different coloured lens this time. It was like the universe had wiped the slate clean, pushed the cosmic reset button and there she was, just like that. A little girl offering me a second chance. Together we could open the door to possibility, the possibility to right past wrongs. She represented the vulnerable little girl in me that longed to be accepted, valued and understood. The little girl in my heart that still in many ways yearned to be her true self, that wanted more than anything to be able to maintain a sense of self-belief and worthiness.

Over the years it had become crystal clear that in many ways I didn't want to become like my own mother. Having a little girl of my own was the push to wake me up and realise that as much as I didn't want to become a version of mum, I didn't want Lola to turn into me either. Not the way that I had been in recent years anyway. I can admit now that my first eight years of motherhood, first with Gabe and then followed by Riley, I *had* become a version of my mum. A workaholic over-achiever, who didn't have time to stop and really *feel*, whose self-worth was definitely wrapped up in how busy and stressed she was on any given day. When Lola came into my life I knew that changing the cycle for my daughter meant I had to start with a further willingness to change things about myself. The shit that no longer served me had to stop.

Like Gabriel, Lola at birth felt old and wise. From the second I clocked eyes on her I was overwhelmed with a sense of "Hi! It's so good to see you again." The feeling was a familiar one, as if we'd known each other before. As if she had showed up in my life to remind me of who I was *really* here to be, to crack me open, to get me well and truly over the line. I must admit that I've never really felt like her mother; much more like her little twin soul. And with her in my life, things felt lighter.

Lola's arrival brought on many different emotions. I felt I had a new chance to do things differently with her and for her, and I became dramatically aware of a new and deep need within my own heart — to create a world where I trusted she would feel safe. I wanted her to grow up and be free from anxiety and self-loathing. I didn't want her to go through the same things I did, and I also did *not* want to end up living vicariously through my daughter later on in life.

Many concerns about raising a little girl began circulating in my mind, but they didn't last long. Taking Lola's lead I quickly learned to give up worrying. It was Lola herself that had it covered. I can't help but laugh out loud when I recall Riley's kindergarten project from a couple of years back paints a picture of Lola's personality so eloquently. He was asked to give a speech on his family. It went like this:

"My dad is the best.
He plays footy with me and turns the music up
super loud when we are in the car.
My mum is really kind, she is fun and caring
and she cooks the best cupcakes.
My brother Gabe is my best friend. I love him.
And then there's Lola. She's my little sister
and she is THE BOSS!"

Far out we laughed until we cried when Riley first recited those words. The truth straight out of the mouth of babes. From the get go she always was little 'Lola Fierce.' At the ripe old age of two it was clear that she was unapologetic in who she would one day become. But at the same time, endlessly sweet, loving, and affectionate, whilst embodying a fire of self-love within. I know, just like her brothers, my little Lolly Dolly (as I call her) joined me on this planet to take my hand and pull me through.

Three years ago I really needed her. I was lost. Again. And anxiety had me reeling once more. How did I know? Because I had slipped back into that familiar feeling. The one where I felt like

I needed to push harder, to hold on, to have all the answers, and to keep it together, to people please and to get everything right. My default switch had flicked on and I was set on all the things I had to *do* for life, instead of focusing on how I needed to be so that life just flowed. I was losing perspective again, and of course at the time I didn't know it. On the surface, don't you worry, my life appeared to be amazing. I had three beautiful children, a successful gym, and I was winning awards and accolades for my community achievements. I had received a lot of press that year, my mummy wellness program was thriving, and we had recently sold one of our start-up concepts — a health-food business we had started with my sister Han. Apparently I was winning at life and everyone kept asking "how do you do it?" We were taking regular overseas holidays as a family, life was amazing yet I was so: Desperately. Unhappy. And so ridiculously done with being unhappy. I couldn't stand myself. Again. Man this shit was getting old.

If I'm honest, I had a huge problem being honest with myself.

I recently learned that the definition of speaking your truth is: "acknowledging *all* that is so for you. Your thoughts, your feelings and your behaviour."

After ten years I was still certainly failing to fully acknowledge *all* of what was so for me. I was resistant to speaking my truth. I was also still dwelling in the shadows of shame, incredibly frightened of judgement. I withheld a part of myself, I withheld the whole truth about my struggle for self-acceptance in the face of my long-term battle with anxiety. The dark stigma of mental illness enveloped my entire being, and that fear in so many ways kept me from telling the whole story. The whole story was that my mental breakdown had completely catapulted my life into this direction, *because* of my illness I had become who I was, but because of the shame I remained resistant to seeing it that way. I worried a lot about people finding out about my mental health history. And I didn't feel comfortable sharing my story with anyone outside of my immediate family or close circle of friends. In my Mums Empowered work I referenced postnatal depression because I believed that to be much more relatable, more widely accepted, and of course it gave new mothers hope that they too could climb back to health and a positive mindset. But my chronic anxiety, psychosis, schizophrenia prognosis, and the time I spent locked away in mental hospitals? Well all *that* made me 'crazy', fragile and unreliable. Perhaps even dangerous.

All of a sudden the self-judgement was next level, and therefore the truth about my past was locked away. Try as I might — I couldn't find the key.

You can hit a lot rock bottoms in life. And rock bottom can look different for everyone. For me, it came in the form of an electrical storm that swept through our home town.

I didn't see my crash coming, but I did know that something wasn't quite right. It was like the continuous feeling that the picture needs to clock an inch or so to be straight. I just got a sense that something was not quite right, but at the time I never thought to turn inward and question the anxiety in my gut that was playing its all too familiar tune. Surely by now I *knew* the first port of call was to be kind to myself. But no. Instead, I did the opposite. I looked to the external circumstances of my life, the situations I felt I could somehow control, I blamed other people as the reasons why I felt incomplete and uneasy. With my default switch activated, I came up with the usual answer. I obviously wasn't *doing* enough. I needed to *do* more. And in doing more I would feel like I was enough and I'd find peace. Right?

Oh, hell to the no! I couldn't have been further from right. I ended up with bacterial pneumonia. I was so removed from my own body that I actually had had pneumonia for about four weeks without even realising it. I eventually became so physically ill resulting in permanent scarring on my left lung, but with pneumonia unbeknown to me, I just kept doing what I thought I had to do. I kept pushing through,

I didn't have time to be sick, which clearly said a lot about the path I was treading.

Cue the huge electrical storm. We lost power in our suburb for a week. Considering that a large portion of the world's population lives without electricity, the situation was not a big deal in comparison. Surely I could keep it together. Apparently absolutely not. The loss of power was the catalyst that saw me lose power too, and it became perfectly evident to me, to Jase and to my kids that this time, I was not coping with life. Seriously not coping. Ever since my psychotic breakdown, which was at this point ten years ago, I'd never really felt like I wasn't actually coping. I always coped. I ate well. I exercised. I worked hard. I did my best. I was always okay. I managed. I got up. I pushed through. I got on with it. But during the storm, I literally had to go to bed, I couldn't deal. At one point, Jase sat on the end of the bed with a look of worry that I'd never seen on his face before. He knew that this time it was a little different. I was not in a good place. On one hand I was so angry at the world, and on the other so deeply resentful of myself. The all too familiar frustration arose again as the self-questioning loop thoughts of "why can't I cope?" and "what is wrong with me?" circulated on repeat in my mind like a broken record. I was living a privileged life, and the power had gone out for a moment. Big fucking deal. How dare I be so ungrateful and miserable?!

I remember having a conversation with Jason a couple of weeks before the storm in an attempt to articulate the fact that something didn't feel right, yet I couldn't quite put my finger on what it was. I stumbled to find the words.

*"I feel like I'm not my whole self,
like people don't truly know the real me."*

Jase didn't have to think about his response.
He was angry.

*"You need to get over yourself! You are being absolutely ridiculous. Don't you understand? Your life cannot thrive on what other people think of you, it's up to you to not withhold your wholeself regardless of what others may or may not think. Who gives a shit. And besides all of that Em, you've just been named
as a finalist in the god damn Steel Magnolia Awards* (an honourable award presented by a reputable charity). *That accolade is not an easy one to achieve, it takes guts and grit and determination. It is greatly symbolic of your contribution and efforts as a woman of generosity and strength! Is that not enough to make you realise that people fucking understand you? What more could you possibly want Em?!"*

He was so worked up, and even through his confrontation and frustration, he was imploring me to see the light. But I dug my heels in and blatantly refused. This time my anxiety was my muse. I clung to it. In the end Jase threw up his hands.

"I really don't know what else you want Em. You want the impossible. You are never good enough for you. And that shit is getting old."

I had completely lost sight of telling *my* truth, that it's ok to not always have it together, that no one ever really does have it all worked out. That my anxious mind and history of breakdown wasn't necessarily a personal curse, but a reality that many people come up against every day. Instead of immersing myself in the lessons I had learned since my breakdown and drawing upon them to help others, I was labelling, comparing and judging. Playing the part and the 'fake it till you make it' card to the best of my ability. Well I certainly wasn't making it. I was goddamn losing it.

I was so hung up on this idea that people weren't understanding the real me. When I finally realised the problem was that I actually wasn't *showing them* the real me. Liz Gilbert, although I've never met her, had the perfect words to describe the real me,

"a glorious mess."

Yep there I was. One huge glorious mess.

Even through my anxiety and all of the ups and downs and round and rounds, in my life I have been extremely blessed. I've been fortunate. I've been successful in my career, people have tended to like me, I have had a beautiful network of love and support around me, and I had managed to keep my family somewhat functioning. Yet there I was remaining to be so unkind and downright cruel toward myself. I was resistant to loving myself, whilst consistently expecting more from myself. I was refusing to show-up amidst the shame, I was not prepared to expose myself as imperfect and vulnerable, and you know — slightly nuts. A part of me was hiding, a piece of the puzzle missing, and no one could ever complete it but me. If I wasn't happy, the buck stopped with me. I longed to be authentic and genuine and true to myself. But I wasn't exactly sure where to start. I felt like I was back at the beginning. A very good place to start apparently. Cue an anxiety-fueled mini-breakdown to kick things off post electrical storm.

I existed merely in body as the mind was definitely fragile. It was intense, and strangely at the time I wasn't able to recognise the symptoms as anxiety. Off and on throughout my life I've always managed to come up with a myriad of excuses for my non-stop thinking, for my intensity, for the constant questioning of my thoughts and feelings, for my continuous jitters, and for my desperate need to remain on guard. Forget elephants, anxiety was a long-time beast in the room, and the time was fast approaching to tame that fucking wild cat once and for all.

I didn't know what to do with the kids at that time. I remember standing there in the kitchen with a torch, staring at the wall feeling completely helpless. The fact that I couldn't boil water to make a cup of tea meant my life was over. I was beyond stressed and ridiculously negative. I called my girlfriend whose home had not been affected by the power outage and she immediately heard the strain in my voice. She quickly welcomed us over. On auto-pilot I was able to cook us a hot meal on her stove, I bathed the kids and we recharged our phones. The luxury of a few hours of electricity was bliss and it really helped to take the edge off my completely unrelated nerves. I really didn't want to worry my friend or to have her see the truth of how much I was struggling, so I put my brave face on and did my best to present as usual, you know, as if I had it altogether.

She could see straight through it and I couldn't keep kidding myself either.

Jason was getting concerned. "It's only power babe. It's going to come back on. I think you're overreacting, you should try and get out of bed." He kept saying it to me. But no matter how hard I tried I just couldn't keep anything in perspective. I had totally lost my energy and it had zero to do with the loss of electricity. The only answer was to stay in bed.

Of all the times it could have occurred, it was the following weekend, still without power, that Jase and I had an important meeting booked to attend interstate with a new business coach. We were planning on exploring the idea of franchising and expanding our Mums Empowered business. This was a huge step, and having that bubbling away in the background was certainly a contributor to my anxiety. This particular business coach had a wonderful reputation for knowing her stuff, she could offer years of experience and guidance in making sure the business model and brand was watertight; ultimately you had to 'qualify' to be taken on as her client. Of course, I was riddled with fear which prompted me to play out a whole dire scenario in my mind... I would walk into the meeting and she would look me up and down and say,

"Welcome basket case,

now just what the hell is your deal?

You are so far from having what it takes.

Why are you here wasting my time?!"

There I was self-loathing again in spades, lying there with the sheets pulled up over my ears, imagining all the different ways this meeting could go horribly wrong. Like usual I was making sure to lay the extra pressure on. Because you know, that's helpful.

The kids were supposed to be heading to their grandparent's place for the weekend but in the end, they too had no electricity and therefore couldn't babysit. This provided me with yet another opportunity to be stressed and anxious and overwhelmed. I decided the whole thing wasn't meant to be, it was all too hard. I wanted to cancel the meeting and stay in bed.

Jase took control. He was all for forging ahead despite the various difficulties standing in the way, namely myself of course, so the kids came with us for the weekend. I remember sitting on the plane thinking, "why the hell are we doing this?" This time I recognised the ground beneath my feet was shaky and I didn't pretend that it wasn't. I was in the grip of anxiety and I couldn't find a way out. In the end, I was so thankful the little ones were there. Forcing me to stay present and attend to their immediate needs helped me to feel grounded. I didn't trip all the way over the edge.

Jason loved the initial meeting, because the business coach was fierce. She was an excellent saleswoman and she didn't hold back in telling me, "you need to get it together Em. You must be prepared to stand up and believe in yourself. Trust me honey, I eat women like you for breakfast, and *that* is why I am successful." She had a certainty about her that I found intimidating and confrontational. My sensitivity was activated and almost immediately I began beating myself up for being too soft. The meeting lasted an intense four hours, I gritted my teeth the whole time and managed to hold it together until the end. That afternoon I almost collapsed from exhaustion. I felt so pressured that we had signed the contract on the spot, and none of it felt right. Riddled with self-doubt I couldn't find the words to speak for myself and make the decision that felt right in my heart. The right decision would have been to admit how I was feeling right there and then, the truth was I was struggling to breathe let alone think clearly. I was not fit mentally nor physically to make any kind of business calls. I needed space and time, and I gave myself neither.

We were staying at my friend's house. I paced the guest bedroom berating myself for having landed back in this frustrating place of total overwhelm. There was a strange familiarity in the air surrounding me, it took me straight back to the time when I was 20 in the lead up to my breakdown. That frightened me. I couldn't afford to go back there. Yet there I was, treading those same waters again. I was heavy with resentment for being back in this dark mental place, and I was so god damn sick of myself. Children were starving on this planet for gods sake, yet there I was torturing myself over first world problems. Around and around the merry go round I went until I was literally overcome with physical pain in my head and in my gut. I was silent screaming, "I'm sick of myself. Please help me." All of a sudden I realised I was on my knees praying, "Please help me. I surrender. I'll do whatever it is that you want me to do. Please set my mind free." I didn't even consider who or what I was praying to, but I had desperately given up the control. I felt frustrated and stupid and self-righteous and spoilt and guilty. I had a beautiful life, with so many blessings, why couldn't I cope? Why wasn't I happy? What was there not to like? What was wrong with me?

The more questions I asked, the more panicked I became. I was doubled over clutching my stomach, gasping for air as I knelt there. I knew

I could no longer do this on my own. It was a case of surrender. I said the words out loud, "Dear God, I will not survive if I don't change this now. I can't keep playing this worst enemy bullshit game with myself any longer. I am sick of being so serious all of the time. Help me to get over myself. Please use me, I want to be able to serve others, I want to get over myself." The tears streamed down my face and I was too defeated to even wipe them away. I couldn't get up; it felt like the entire weight of my life, my past, my future, was pressing down on my back.

That's when I felt it. Still on my knees as I silently wept, I felt two hands gently bear down on my shoulders. It was such a shock as I was sure I was alone, I hadn't heard anyone sneak into the room. I turned around, and there was no one there. I can't even begin to tell you what it felt like — as I climbed carefully to my feet I should have been frightened. But I wasn't, not at all. Instead I had this overwhelming sense of a presence standing with me, the air in the room was different and the feeling in that moment gave me immediate comfort. Now I know it sounds crazy, and given my history, I don't blame you for wondering if I'd somehow triggered the onset of a psychotic break. But this was not insanity. I knew *in my bones* there was nothing woo-woo about it, and

> I knew in a way that I hadn't known before,
> everything was going to be okay.

I woke up the next day and the ground had
stopped shaking, anxiety had left the building.
My mind had stopped racing and I finally felt
relieved, but holy shit was I tired. About an hour
before we were due to leave for the airport
and return home, the business coach who
had chaired our killer meeting the day before
knocked on the door. As I went to greet her she
reached into her handbag and removed from it
a book. The book was thick and looked heavy,
it had a dark navy-blue cover and sprawled
in gold lettering across the cover read
A Course in Miracles.

*"I sat up in bed in the middle of the night with
a feeling that I should give this to you."*
She held the book out to me with two hands.

I smiled back at her. *"Wow. Thank you so much for the
offer, but actually I don't need that."*

She frowned, slightly confused. *"Oh. I really felt
that you did need it. Are you sure you don't want it?*

Do you even know what this is? Have you read it already?"
It became obvious to me that she actually didn't
know herself what she was giving to me.

I shut the door behind us as we stepped into the
white tiled entry hall. *"Yes, I know what it is, and no I
have not read it. But I also know I don't want to read it, nor
do I need it right now. My mother is a student of the Course
and has been for years. Maybe one day I'll study it, but now
is not the time. I'm not ready. Thanks anyway though."*
Little did I know I was completely intercepting
an act of grace.

She put the book back in her bag. *"Okay.
Fair enough then. I haven't read it myself,
what's it all about?"* She looked curious.

I folded my arms and lead her into the kitchen.
*"Basically, it's a spiritual curriculum, one of many different
types that exist, comprising universal or metaphysical
truths. I really do have a very limited understanding of it
though, so I'm probably best not to comment."*

"Rightio then." She seemed interested.
*"Are you absolutely certain you don't want
the book? I really did feel compelled to pass
it on to you."*

"Positive. No thank you." I was certain.
And that was just the beginning.

194.

You see there was a reason why I rejected the offer of this book. My mother was a long-time student of *A Course of Miracles*, she had first picked it up at least twenty years ago or more, probably when I was around 12 years old. Mum intellectualised everything within its pages, and the book would almost literally steal her away from us. I remembered as a child her discussing the spiritual concepts within its pages and I had found it incredibly confusing, abstract and almost frightening at times. For almost days at a time she would be distant and lost in thought. There was a time there that it was all she ever wanted to talk about and although I longed to understand her fascination, as a struggling teen I just wanted my mum to *be* there. In many ways I resented it. Off the back of feeling like I lost my mother to the *Course*, the use of Christian terminology throughout its pages meant I absolutely renounced religion and religious practice of any kind.

In follow up to my business development strategy, not long after that weekend away I engaged in an 'unconscious values test'. Interestingly it was discovered through the test (which consisted of a series of questions each requiring one solid answer), that my highest value in life was Spirituality. This came as a shock. Surprisingly, the least important value in my life according to the test was Physical Health. I cracked up laughing, was someone playing a trick on me? After all, I had spent the last good part of a decade focusing on physical health. Then the penny dropped and I began to realise the results of the test actually made a lot of sense. No wonder over the years I had felt continuously uncomfortable and out of alignment working within the fitness industry where the focus is solely on physicality. It turned out that the career path I was on *was* fairly incongruent with my unconscious values.

I had always known in my heart that my passion and interest in fitness in fact came from my experience with mental illness, and how I had personally lived and breathed the benefits of physical exercise to change my mental state, to help ease depression and anxiety. All I wanted to do was to help others, but my long term moral conflict with the industry itself continued to make me feel stuck. Was there a way I could put this right? I started to wonder whether I could be represented or marketed in a different light within the same industry? I had to either change my values and shape myself to fit the current mould, or cut the bullshit and finally show up as the whole me. Spirituality and all. There were choices to be made.

Almost immediately I made them. I firstly made a commitment to honour and permit my highest of values. I had rejected faith as a regular practice in my life for a very long time and feared ever saying the 'G' word out loud for all of the judgement and unfortunate connotations that go with it. But I wasn't going to cop my regular excuses, uncomfortable or not, I went there. I went to God. Nothing like taking a giant leap, which I guess in hindsight is really what faith encompasses. One giant leap. Within days I familiarized myself with Marianne Williamson, the remarkable spiritual leader largely responsible for popularising *A Course in Miracles* in the Western world. After a few short weeks of burying myself in her teachings I had become a raving fan. I mean, a much more peaceful raving fan. My heart was really starting to open up. I devoured Marianne's internationally acclaimed best-seller, *A Return to Love.* The book was no joke stuck to my hand for a time. It provided a simple explanation of the principles of the *Course* and I laughed my way through the pages because I realised at the end of the day she was a seeker just like me. Like Marianne, I had tried everything outside of myself to get the picture hanging straight on the wall and the colours to shine the brightest. Like her I was constantly searching, to the point where I ended up doubled over, landing on my knees feeling invisible hands placed upon my shoulders. I surrendered. And everything began to fall into place.

Reading *A Return to Love* really was my return home. I soon realised that the gaping hole in my life was my faith in a power bigger than myself; there I was thinking I could control everything outside of myself. I had refused to look deep enough within. I had a huge problem. That problem was a God problem. In many ways I was curious, like "what even *is* God?" I had always struggled with the way in which many preach using this G word, and yet how in so many destructive ways on this planet, the whole God and religion thing has separated us. No wonder so many of us have struggled to even say the word, let alone believe. I feel the way in which we use particular words and language to convey our *thinking,* to organise our thought, can ultimately be what divides us. You only need to consider the kind of division that largely occurs between organised religions, to know what I am talking about. Yet at the centre of religion is *faith*, and ironically

faith is so far from organised thinking.

Why do we continuously try and intellectualise what never really can be intellectualised? Faith is beyond thought, it is beyond articulation in words. And from what I have learned, faith requires immense amounts of courage because it is a huge risk that cannot be guaranteed unless you jump right in. You can call it whatever you want to call it, Religion, Spirituality, God, the Universe, Love, Energy...

The truth is, at the heart of it all *is heart*.
And I can't even begin to describe the feeling
of relief that washed over me when I finally
recognised this. It was my "Aha" moment
as Oprah calls it.

My head had forever let me down. Depression and
anxiety were the two main constants in my life
whether I wanted them to be there or not.
They were the cards I was dealt. It was time
I made the commitment, it was time to live
consciously from the heart. I would feel my way
forward. Having always been an avid thinker,
I expected this shift would be a challenge.
Let's face it — I had lived my life up until this point
well and truly caught in my head. My capacity
to think and think fast was what I had deemed
time and time again to be my biggest asset.
Yet I couldn't have been further off the mark.
Plugging in to my spirituality was like taking
one giant breath of fresh air. It was as if I had
forgotten where I lived for a while, and then out
of the blue I remembered the way straight back
to my own front door. It was as if I could fluently
communicate in a foreign language without
any prior training. It was peace like I had never
experienced it before.

Oh man did the flood gates open! Every book
I could read on spirituality I devoured.
I began following incredible heart teachers and
leaders, spiritual greats such as Depak Chopra,
Louise Hay, Eckhart Tolle and Wayne Dyer to

name a few. And finally I felt the time was right to become a student of *A Course in Miracles*.

My newfound faith provided me continued courage to want to step out from behind the façade. I realised that up until this point I had been spruiking a great deal of talk about empowerment and positivity and the journey upward, yet failing to honestly mention the truth about the downs. And at the end of the day, the hole I was constantly seeking to fill since my psychotic breakdown was one I couldn't fill on my own. If I wasn't prepared to admit that — then I knew I would keep on pretending, living day by day behind an iron mask that concealed my shitty sense of constant hopelessness.

Although my head (still stuck in fear) at first said absolutely hell-to-the-no, my heart said it was ok to admit my struggle, to tell my story, to speak of my faith, to lean in. That no matter how frightening the stigma and judgement and self-loathing could be, there were people out there just like me, completely isolated in their mental torture, not realising they are not alone. It was time to accept the fact that I had always been a total headcase and follow my heart.

To know what faith is, you must first know what faith is not.

I knew what it meant to have none, I had lived in faithlessness for long enough.

I took a deep breath and got set for smooth sailing. Right into the biggest shit storm.

PEAS & PORRIDGE

CHAPTER ELEVEN

It was 3am when I sat bolt upright in bed with a stabbing pain cutting through my chest.

I was having a heart attack. Well that's what I thought it was. But it wasn't. It was a panic attack. I'd never really had a full-blown panic attack before. I was crippled with cold, hard fear. The tingles ran up and down my spine scurrying like tiny ants in a production line. My skin crawled. My senses were heightened. The chest pain was intense. I could hear footsteps outside the bedroom door. There was an intruder in the house, poised at any moment ready to attack me. He was right outside, I just knew he was. I was damn certain I wasn't alone.

In reality, I was alone. I wasn't to be the victim of a violent home invasion, but a victim trapped inside my own mind again, with nerves trembling to match. Was I entering psychosis again? I reached for my phone and fumbled with the keypad, I needed to talk to my sister urgently. What time was it in the U.S. anyway? Screw it. I made the call. If it was 3am here that meant it was daytime over there and surely she would pick up the phone.

I was relieved to hear her familiar voice at the end of the line. I was literally at the end of my line. The physical pain was real and I knew once again that I couldn't go on without her. And just like she used to do, when I was 10 years old and had worked myself up into a crazy state, she calmed me down. Speaking all the right words, asking all the right questions, and providing all the right answers. My sister and soul buddy again came to my aid.

My breathing settled. The pain in my heart subsided. My sanity silently returned. No psychosis. There was hope. I made a cup of tea and climbed back into bed as the sun was rising.

A FEW DAYS EARLIER...

**He was different. Something had changed.
I could feel it in my bones.**

Everything appeared normal, the same, nothing out of the ordinary. Yet I felt in my gut something wasn't right.

I tried for months to avoid it. To push the feelings aside, sweep them under the rug and keep powering on. But as each day passed it became more and more obvious that I needed to acknowledge what the hell was going on.

The space between us was widening. We had gone from being peas and carrots to being peas and porridge. We just didn't go together anymore.

I prepared myself for the conversation by rehearsing it over and over *and over* in my mind. And then the thought trickled in: maybe nothing was wrong. Maybe it was all in my head. Maybe I was just losing my mind. Was it all just a figment of my imagination? If it was then I could expect him to say something along the lines of; "Oh Em, what are you even talking about? You have got yourself all worked up and stressed for nothing. Everything is fine, nothing has changed between us."

I would've loved for him to say that, but he didn't say that. Instead what he said was,

"To be honest Em, I don't know how I feel anymore, about you or anything for that matter. I am at the end of my rope with you and I don't know what to do. It's been hard. Really hard. Being married to you is hard."

Could he say hard just one more time? The ground shook beneath my feet. I felt dizzy. I was going to throw up. I had been pacing up and down the street outside my office. I looked around desperately for a place to sit down.

"What do you mean?" I stammered.
"Are you saying that you don't love me?"

Please God. No. I simply can't handle this right now.

"I'm not saying that Em. I just really don't know anything anymore. But what I do know is that you shouldn't need to ask me that question. No matter how shitty you might be feeling, no matter how tough life gets, what matters most is how you feel about you. You know that! Self-Love is what you preach. That's what you should be focusing on right now, how you feel about you, not how I feel about you."

Oh fuck me sideways. The motivational-self-worth speech was about to commence. Well not today. Not on my watch. I had heard enough. I was already under an enormous amount of stress from an incident I could've never had predicted. He could go and get royally fucked.

My thoughts raced, my heart rate soared, my whole body was covered in an itchy sweat. I had to get out. And get out fast.

I drove to the beach and planted my feet in the sand. Time seemed to stand still as I stared out to sea, the waves crashing ferociously on the shore. They were tumultuous that day, a frothy mix of deep green and white, almost violent as if the earth knew the feelings deep within my gut. I felt shattered. Let down. Broken. And angry. I had thought we were solid. Never in a million moons did I expect his love would hesitate. No matter how tough marriage could get, I always assumed he would be there for me. I felt stupid. And really *really* sorry for myself.

There was a huge eruption at home that night. He had said all that he had needed to say earlier that day, and so when I arrived home, there he was sitting on the couch completely evasive and disengaged, his headphones on, flicking through the junk mail catalogues as if the prior conversation had never happened. It was patronising and condescending. My sadness quickly turned to panic. Up went my walls and into the trenches of defence I crawled. I was sick with frustration. Although I had been difficult to live with at times, so had he. Neither one of us was perfect, and marriage had been a challenge, but show me a marriage that doesn't come with an element of challenge! The anxiety quickly became all-out war and I was overcome with resentment.

I left the next day, I just couldn't handle it. All of a sudden I felt locked out in the cold. He wouldn't talk to me at all. He wanted me to focus on me, there was no 'us.' I became a shaking, blubbering ball of a mess. It was a painfully difficult choice to make but I could barely function in the state I was in, let alone take care of the children. I was becoming a basket case whilst he on the other hand, remained calm. The whole time. Stoic. Cold. In control. I didn't want to give him any more ammunition as the 'crazy one.' I had to get away for a few days and it made better sense for me to go. I needed to pull my shit together and I needed to be alone to do just that. It was Saturday morning, I packed a bag and reassured each of the kids that mummy would be back for them on Monday afternoon.

The conversation I had with Gabriel at his bedroom window that morning is one that I will carry in my heart for as long as it still beats. I had said my goodbyes to the kids and of course Riley and Lola had no idea what was

really going on. They thought I had to go to
work and the less they knew at that point, the
better. But Gabe knew what was going on.
In his usual way, he knew the truth unspoken.

I walked to my car parked in our driveway when
I noticed his little silhouette standing at his
bedroom window preparing to watch me
drive away. I turned and walked towards him.
I reached out my hand and touched his through the
black gauze fly screen. Tears rolled down his face.

"You know I'll be back for you."
I choked on the words.

"I know mummy." Gabe replied. *"I'm sad for you mum,
but I want you to know you can get through this. You are
strong enough, it's just that you have forgotten that.
Dad does love you, I know he does. He told me he does. But
right now he feels he can't love anything. So mum, this really
isn't about you. And even though you are sad, you must accept
it. You have to accept him and where he's at, ok?"*

And there amidst my tears that little angel
softly weaved his magic once more. My rock.
The man of my dreams sent to save me,
effortlessly articulating all that I needed to hear

to give me the strength to move forward. I truly had no words. I think I whispered a thank you as I stood there staring back at him from outside the window. I knew he was right. As I pulled my car out of the driveway I didn't look back.

This time rather than drive fearfully away from the pain, I took the wheel of the car and ploughed headfirst into it. Anxiety landed me alone on the timber floor at my mum's city apartment for the best part of three days. She had left town for the weekend and I always kept a key to her front door. I literally passed the time wailing on the kitchen floor, only getting up occasionally to take solace under the heavy white quilt on her bed, the weight of it against my body was secure and comforting. It was there in the early hours of the Sunday morning that I sat bolt upright in bed, literally feeling my heart breaking in two, thinking there was an intruder in the apartment.

"You're ok Em." Pete's soothing voice met my ear from the other end of the phone line. "You can get through this sweetheart. It's just your body responding to the anxiety. Calm down. Yes, you are alone, but trust me, you have nothing to fear. You actually need to be alone right now to be able to process everything. Just breathe for now. Don't get so far ahead of yourself. One moment at a time. Ok darling." Hearing those words was like aloe vera on sun scorched skin.

As my breathing slowed, a significant realisation came to mind. I realised in over 30 years I had never ever spent any more than a few hours completely on my own. It was like I constantly needed the stimulation of others to sustain myself. I needed to feel needed, and I needed continual reassurance. I realised I was still grossly dependent upon the approval of other people in order to be ok. At 4.00am as I crept into the tiny kitchen to make my cup of tea, being all by myself brought me a renewed sense of comfort. I wasn't lonely, I was alone. And I was *meant* to be alone. This silver lining was the perfect opportunity to search my soul in ways I'd never done before. I prayed to God for help, I prayed to be shown my darkness, and I prayed to know my light. Then I sat in silence before getting out my journal and I wrote, and I wrote, and I wrote.

What you probably need to know is that a few months prior to this weekend vigil of solitude, the year had started on an all-time high. In alignment with the solid decisions I'd made the previous year — to be my wholehearted self, to share my story and to pursue a career helping others along their mental wellness journeys, Jase and I finally made the call to sell our gym. It was a huge call. We'd been in business for almost a decade, and the place had become a family institution. Both Riley and Lola were born and raised on that rubber floor surrounded by kettle bells and Pilates mats. The fact was Jason's personal career was taking him away from the physical fitness space too, landing him further down the holistic healing track. And I was super keen to pursue my work with youth, delivering emotional intelligence education to high school students, whilst leading empowerment programs for women and communities. I had successfully acquired an equity partner in my new business venture, and there was no looking back. It was all green for go. We had to tie up the loose ends and move on. I was fairly unemotional at the time, business was business. I was looking ahead and I was ready to launch. Um, well at least I thought I was.

I noticed the shudder breathing well before I actually understood what was happening. You know how when small children are really upset, they take those short, succinct, little breaths all in a row to calm down? Well, apparently, they're called shudder breaths. And out of nowhere I started breathing like that *all* of the time. No tears. No apparent stress or anxiety. Just shudder breathing. It was weird and I brought it up in conversation with Peta.

"I'm doing this weird breathing thing." I told her.
"Like I would if I was a little girl and I was really upset, attempting to calm myself down through my tears. But I

don't feel sad or emotional at all. It's so bizarre.
I'm going to give up caffeine and see if that helps."

"Maybe the little girl inside of you is really upset."
She replied straight off the bat
"Perhaps there's a part of you that is really really sad.
But you've been too busy all this time to notice her."

I responded with an uncomfortable laugh.
How could I be sad? I certainly didn't feel sad.
Was I really missing the point? Could she be right?

Everything seemed to be soaring, the picture
was pretty much straight on the wall. I decided
to cut back on the caffeine for a while and
leave it at that.

Of course, in hindsight, I wished I paid more
attention to those itty-bitty repetitive shudder
breaths. They literally were the only prior
warning for the shit storm that I was on route
to directly encounter.

It was a shit storm that saw me successfully
preview the original manuscript of this very
book to a sell-out audience, only to never be
able to publish it. It was the shit storm that saw

me expose the skeletons in my closet in a very public way, turning the 'fit mum who had her crap together' analogy well on its head, only to feel like a right royal attention-seeking fucktard for having spoken up about mental illness.

It was the shit storm that saw me re-write and change the title of this book only a mere three times. It was the shit storm that landed me in my solicitor's office and saw me instantly lose a close friend, colleague and confidant, who meant more to me than we both knew at the time. It was the shit storm that saw me lose thousands of dollars, lose my hair, lose my dignity, almost lose my marriage, and most definitely lose my faith for a time. It was the shit storm that left me buried in shame, face down in a pile of shit, eating shit, smelling like shit. I think you get the point.

And that's where I remained for nine months. Not just buried in shame, frozen in it. I couldn't move. I couldn't speak. I couldn't even scream. I was in a deep hole. It had been more than a decade since I'd contemplated taking my own life, I thought about it more so than anything else during that shit storm. I hid from the world. And I hated the world. I binge watched Netflix. And I stopped praying. 'G' became the capital for Gin, and gin only. I was having a right old pity party, balloons and all. Once again the ultimate victim of circumstance, helpless, powerless, a total fraud. The imposter entered the chambers of my mind. The torment of anxiety circulated, swooped and smothered me crowding all of my senses.

"Look at your kids Em" Jase was determined to help me. "Draw your energy from them. What do you want them to know about life? That it's easy? Or that at times it's really tough, but you *can* get through it. You just gotta stick together and ride it out. You're allowed to be upset. It is unfair. But when does it come a time that enough

He was being a motivational speaker again, but in many ways —he was right. I knew no one ever said life was going to be easy, nor did they say it would be fair. The advice my dad gave me as a young child came flooding back, "the only thing you can control in this life Em is how you choose to respond to things as they happen." It was my response-ability that mattered the most now. I had lay down for long enough. I didn't want to be a victim anymore. I looked back at what had happened, the ultimate cause of the shit storm, with a determination this time to hold the mirror up and look at myself. What was it I *needed* to learn?

First I looked at my darkness. I learned that in wading into the discomfort of telling my story,

I had triggered my default switch — I always sidestepped to avoid the whole truth. Because the whole truth was painful. The whole truth was *I didn't believe in myself*. Without noticing it, perfectionism had taken hold again. I was avoiding walking until I could run. I was holding back until I was 'ready', people pleasing again, seeking approval and attention and saying yes when I really wanted to be saying no. Lesson on repeat much? I was fucking exhausted but I didn't put the mirror down. I kept staring into it, determined to break the cycle of my usual self-sabotage. *I needed to know my light.*

Weeks past, I had a few lame attempts at joining in on life but I wasn't really getting anywhere, the anxiety just wouldn't subside. I had to simplify, get back to basics. First step was dealing with the chronic anxiousness in my body, which meant considering my diet and sleep quality. I was struggling with both and putting my physical heath last was not winning me any favours mentally and emotionally. I made dramatic changes in my lifestyle habits, giving up alcohol and coffee and eating mainly a plant-based diet. I stopped high impact exercise, trading it for deep breathing sessions instead. I meditated. Even when it felt impossible to sit still, I meditated. I read. I walked. I sat in the sun. I played with the kids. I lowered my expectations. I prayed. I was kinder to myself.

And by no means was any of it easy.

There were times where following through on my commitment to becoming healthier felt more difficult and confronting than the actual anxiety itself. My nervous system was definitely grateful, it began to let go as I embraced the simple life. I celebrated the little wins like being able to remain in my lane when a loud motorcycle passed by my driver's window, or waking up in the morning having actually slept a whole eight hours as opposed to having lay there all night with my eyes closed pretending, whilst my body buzzed with adrenaline as if I had a finger in a power point. The lifestyle changes were definitely paying off. Body, mind and soul.

Without the constant buzz of busy I had more time to just be. More time to think about the state of my life, who I was, what I liked, what I wanted and what I stood for. In this new state of 'be-ing' I came to one very confronting conclusion; I didn't know myself very well. At all. I had completely lost myself. How was it that I could possibly not know who the hell I was, when all I had ever wanted was to be the real me? You'd think surely I would have had a clue by now. But I didn't, and there was a reason why I didn't.

The answer hit me straight between the eyes. My entire sense of stability came from others. That meant that the formation of my self-worth was completely in the hands of other people. I had given those around me far too much responsibility, a task that in fact no one could ever achieve for me. I had lived a life up until this point where I hadn't constructed any clear boundaries around what I would and wouldn't accept. I avoided speaking up about what was on my heart for fear of judgment. All because being liked was more important. My impossible expectations always resulted in confusion, resentment, and eventually you guessed it, crippling anxiety.

I had people in my life that never really were my tribe, some of whom I was forced to let go of painfully. And I experienced anguish because I took everything so fucking seriously. I second guessed myself daily, and in the end, I had stood by and watched another year of my life float up shit creek because I was too god damn afraid once again to take a stand and love the whole me. I had been living at effect, unwilling to look deeper at the cause. And trust me, whilst living at effect you are constantly weathering the storm. You eventually do feel powerless and helpless and completely useless. You keep hustling to change the circumstances outside of yourself, yet frustratingly nothing ever changes. No matter what you do. That was me. Every. Single. Day.

Time passed and the self-loathing kept rising to the surface, but I was determined to keep staring into that mirror. I was not going to distract myself or look away this time.

In the darkness, I took a deep breath out and I prayed to be able to know her, to trust her, to be her, the real me. And that was when I saw her looking back at me. There she was, a compassionate, free spirited, determined and deeply sensitive little girl desperate to be free from the persona of weakness that was keeping her bound. She had been forgotten long ago, perhaps in a desperate act of survival. Hiding herself away behind a shiny steel façade had become her safety net. Whilst remaining at the mercy of others at least she knew how the story would play out. With certainty she could always predict how it would end, before the cycle began again. And again. And again.

I stared back at that sweet little cherub and I promised her that she was going to be free. She could put down her shield as there was nothing to defend against anymore. No more victim. She had won. And in victory, she could now take the leap of faith into the unknown, knowing in her heart that whilst ever she loved, embraced, and fully accepted all that she was, she would be safe.

Funnily enough, the proverbial shit storm ended how it started. Me. Tears. On the cold hard kitchen floor. But this time the scene was a little different. Something was missing, something had gone. The little victim version of me, powerless and full of blame, who'd clung on so tightly for all of those years, she had finally left the building. I knew it was time to let go of her. In my heart I'd created this persona because I needed her, but the truth was I simply didn't need her anymore. I wanted to break the cycle. Re-write the story. Change the ending. In simpler terms one might say

I finally grew up.

And oh boy was it time. I put my big girl pants on, determined the boundaries, chose to love myself first, and I grew the hell up.

In growing up I realised that shit happens. It happens to us every day of our lives. Suffering is the human condition, it's the common thread that weaves the tapestry of our connectedness, it's the foundation of our humanity. You simply can't get through life without struggle. But my biggest learning is that it's how you *choose to respond* to the struggle, with love and forgiveness — *that* is the key to transcending your pain. It's not easy but this choice will either slip you into your very own pair of ruby red slippers and lead you home, or have you stuck and weighed down in a fuck-off-heavy pair of concrete boots.

I made my choice. I chose to no longer see

my struggle with mental illness as a weakness, but in fact my greatest strength. For it alone has given me the capacity to help others in a way I never ever thought I could. It is through relatability that I can be of service, having lived through my experience, I now can relate to others who need relatability the most. Mental illness can be isolation, but I eventually chose connection instead. Connection within myself first — belonging to ME, and then to others. I now work hard to offer opportunities of connection to the world as I know with every part of me that 'together' really is how we heal.

At the end of the day, when all is said and done,

I decided ruby red was more my colour and I slipped into those sleek little heels and walked on.

Life now you might ask? Well having finally reached 'Destination Self-Acceptance' I think I want to stay here a while. And just exhale. There are many more destinations to reach though, that's why they call it a journey, or in my terms — one crazy mofo of a ride. And it is one ride I'm forever grateful to still be on. I know one of the best things that's come of my ride so far is my now willingness to live without fear or regret. I took a chance and changed the meaning behind my 'insanity'. If the price of insanity meant I finally remembered this goddamn wild heart, then baby it was worth it. The heart is where I get to live now and it's where I choose to stay. Without suffering who would I be? I guess you could say I just wouldn't be me. And the truth is, there's no one else I want to be.

In keeping true to the times I'll close with my fave insta-meme of the decade:

"I stopped waiting for the light at the end of the tunnel and lit that bitch up myself."

Watch this space...

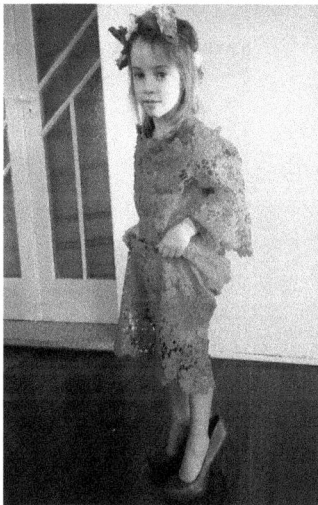

Lola wearing my dress and shoes, 2018

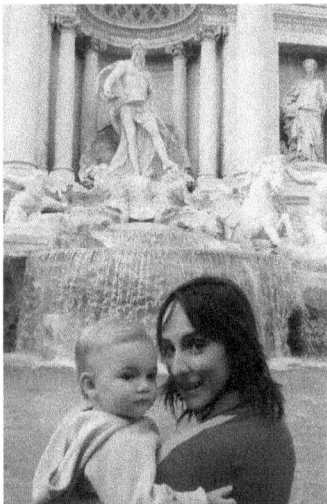

Gabriel and I in Rome, 2007

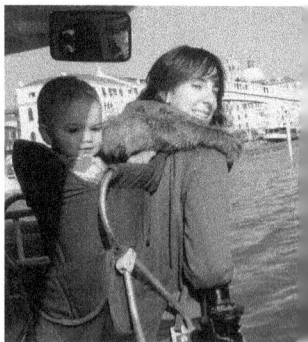

Gabriel and I in Venice, 2007

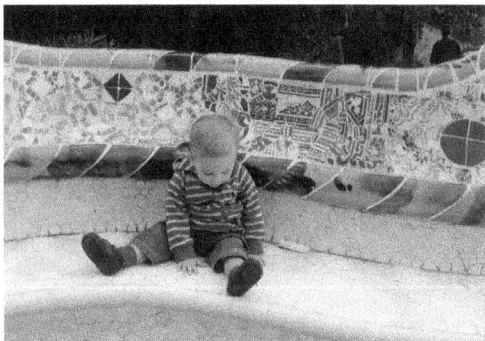

Baby Gabe in Barcelona, 2007

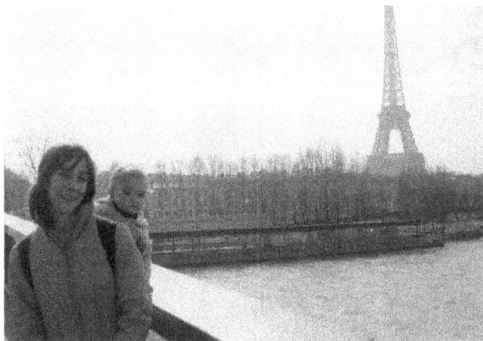

Gabriel and I in Paris, 2007

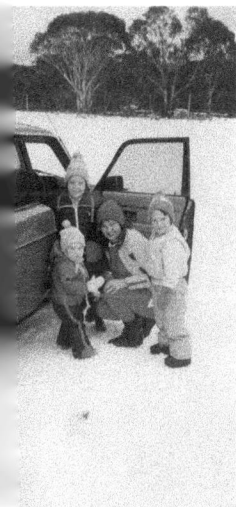

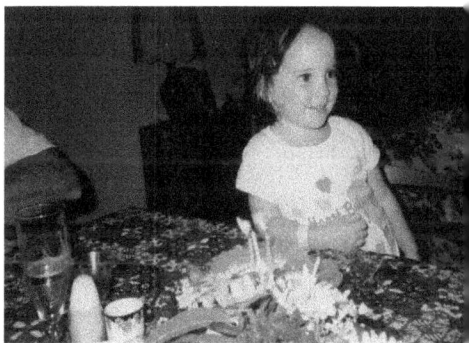

My third birthday, 1987

In the snow with
mum and my sisters, 1988

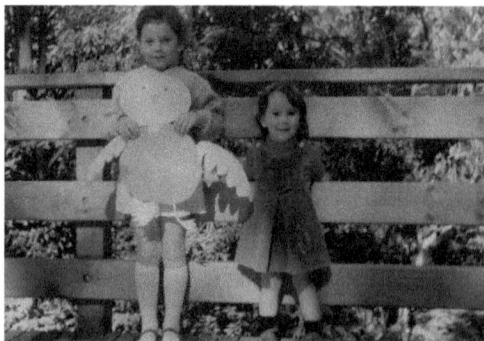

Peta and I aged 6 and 2, 1986

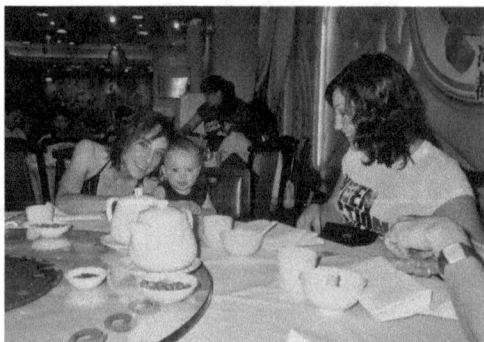

Out for dinner with Gabriel
aged 7 mnths, 2005

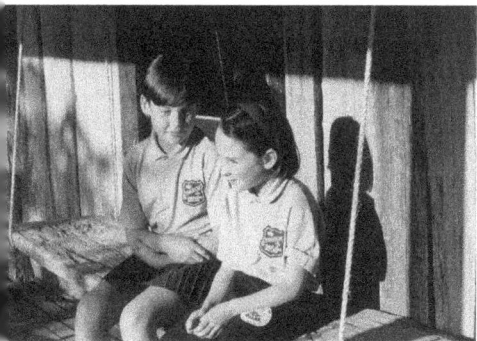

Peta and I in the school yard
at our little Catholic School, 1990

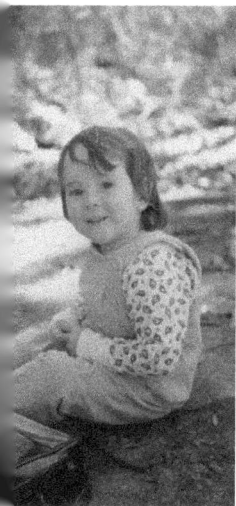

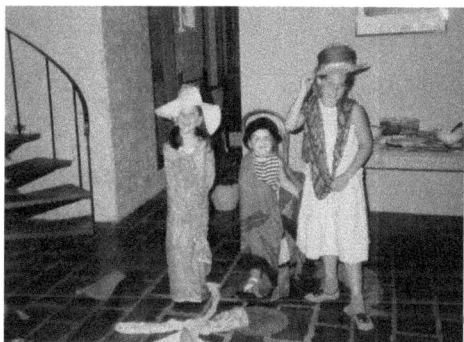

Peta, Hanna and I
playing dress ups, 1992

Me at age 2½, 1986

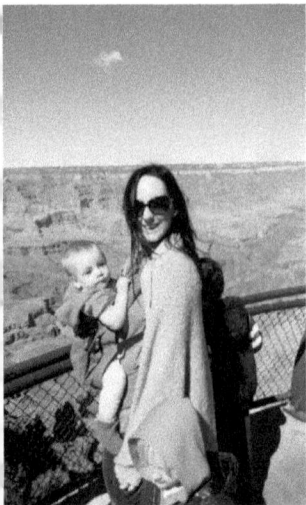

Riley, Lola and I at the
Grand Canyon, A.Z, 2014

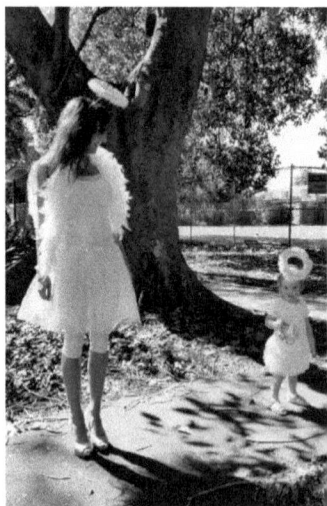

Lola and I dressed up as Angels
for my best friend Abby's 30th
birthday, 2015

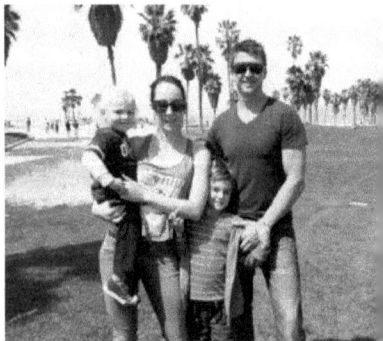

Jose, Gabe, Riley and I
in California, 2012

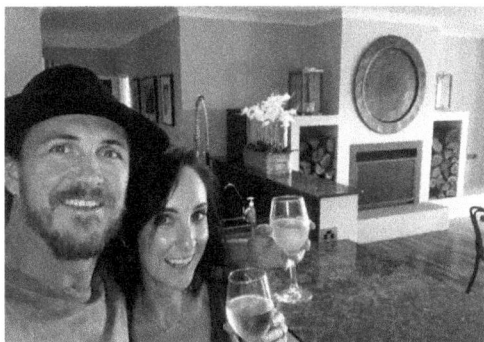

Jase and I in the Hunter Valley, NSW, 2018

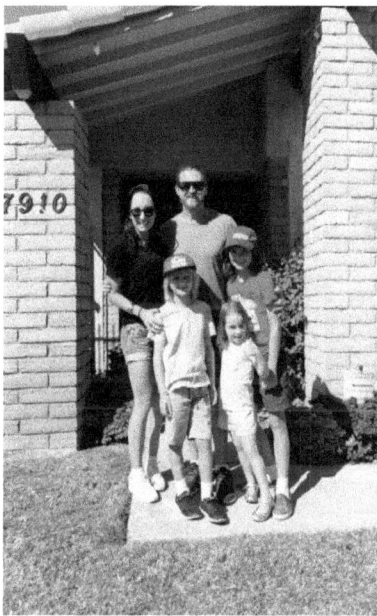

The family in Phoenix, A.Z, 2017

WHERE TO FROM HERE

Em is now dedicated to the prevention of mental illness, and shares her experience and personal story publicly to raise awareness for mental health. She leads and facilitates workshops for schools, workplaces and community groups that promote emotional intelligence, resilience skills, healthy relationships and the art of self-love.

Read more about Em's life and work and download her Top Five Tips for a Whole & Happy Life at: www.emisforyou.com.au

HELP & RESOURCES

If you or anyone you know needs immediate mental health assistance please contact:

Lifeline Australia
Call: 13 11 14
lifeline.org.au

Sane Australia
Call: 1800 18 SANE (7263)
sane.org

Beyond Blue
Call: 1300 224636
beyondblue.org.au

PeriNatal Anxiety and Depression Association (PANDA)
Call: 1300 726 306
panda.org.au

The Butterfly Foundation for Eating Disorders
Call: 1800 334 673
thebutterflyfoundation.org.au

ACKNOWLEDGMENTS

There are so many people to thank and I know that I'd be here for the next year if I was to name everyone individually. I'll start with my children. Gabriel, Riley and Lola. The absolute lights of my life. I wouldn't be who I am today without them having chosen me as their mother. To Jase, my greatest teacher, thank you for helping me see my light. To my father for his boundless love and support, your perspective on life is nothing short of inspirational, thank you for being you. To my mother who has been my rock and one incredible soul buddy the entire way, you were definitely meant for me. To my little sister Han, your sparkle literally lights up so many lives and I am forever grateful that I of all people get to be one of your sisters. To Pete, my best friend and the person who has known the real me the whole time and never ever given up on me regardless of how insane it's been at times, I love you and I cannot thank you enough for being you. To Jay for inspiring me to just do my 'one thing.' It was definitely fate that sat us on that plane side by side. To Carly for saying yes to the constant array of mediocre tasks whilst always keeping the bigger picture in sight, your support in my work means the world. And to Adam for believing in me and this crazy brain that goes with it, you are responsible for turning this dream into a reality and I am eternally grateful. Thank you. To the incredible women in my life who are my constant source of support, energy and encouragement. You know who you are, you are always by my side, you cheer the loudest, and you say all the right things even when it hurts to hear them. The sisterhood in my experience is alive and well. Thank you.

TESTIMONIALS

"Thank you for your memoir. Never in my life, even after all the medication and psychological treatment, have I felt like I can be more than my diagnosis. I have cried more tears than can be imagined tonight but they come from a place of great hope. In a place of such darkness, I can see that there is light, somewhere, if I put the work in. Thank you from the bottom of my heart."
-Jessie

"I wanted to thank you for your memoir, you write with such honesty. Your book has helped me to gain a better understanding of psychosis for which I am grateful. You have touched a stranger's heart and helped make her life a little better. Thank you Em"
- Tracy

"Thank you for the privilege of reading your story. I cried at page 2 and quite a few more times right up to the last page. Thank you for your insight into a different aspect of mental health, one we don't often hear about. You have certainly helped me to look at things differently now. The world is a better place for you being in it."
-Jenni

www.ingramcontent.com/pod-product-compliance
Lightning Source LLC
Chambersburg PA
CBHW060035030426
42334CB00019B/2341